T0361685

CRISIS AND CHAOS

Lessons from the Front Lines of the War Against COVID-19

FORMER SURGEON GENERAL
JEROME M. ADAMS, MD, MPH
WITH NANCY PESKE

POST Hill PRESS

A POST HILL PRESS BOOK
ISBN: 979-8-88845-106-9
ISBN (eBook): 979-8-88845-107-6

Crisis and Chaos:
Lessons from the Front Lines of the War Against COVID-19
© 2023 by Jerome M. Adams, MD, MPH
All Rights Reserved

Cover design by Jim Villaflores

This is a work of nonfiction. All people, locations, events, and situation are portrayed to the best of the author's memory.

Post Hill Press
New York • Nashville
posthillpress.com

Published in the United States of America
1 2 3 4 5 6 7 8 9 10

To my wife, Lacey, and my kids, Caden, Eli, and Millie—
thank you for your love and support.

To all who lost their lives or health to COVID-19 and
to all who did their best to protect others during this
once-in-a-century pandemic, this book was written in
the hopes that your suffering can help prevent the future suffering of others.

CONTENTS

PREFACE

MENTION WASHINGTON, DC, AND MANY people think of out-of-touch insiders focused only on building their power and advancing their own agendas—or they think of a place where their representatives fight for them against those "other people" who are determined to destroy America. Maybe some think of DC as a place where good people do their best to make America live up to its ideals. Growing up in rural, Southern Maryland, I gave little thought to Washington, DC, until my first time there when I was eight years old. Most kids who grew up in the "DMV" (the DC, Maryland, Virginia area) went to the nation's capital on field trips to drive past the White House and see the monuments or to visit the Air and Space Museum. My first visit was for a very different reason. I went there because I was dying. Literally. I was in status asthmaticus, a state where I couldn't breathe. My local hospital—a rural, critical-access hospital forty-five minutes from my house—couldn't reverse the severe asthma attack I was having, so a helicopter airlifted me to the children's hospital, two hours away. Other than confusion, fear, and wondering if I was ever going to see my parents or my dog, Bruno, again, I don't remember much about that day. The idea of a first helicopter ride would normally be exciting for any child, but all I could focus on was not dying, channeling all the energy in my scrawny eight-year-old body into taking each successive breath.

Despite experiencing what many would describe as a traumatic experience, I realize now how lucky I was. Far too many children don't make it to adulthood after such an episode, particularly if they are poor, Black, or living in a rural area (all three describe me as a kid). Black boys die from asthma at three times the rate of White children. Too many live in environments that lead to or worsen their asthma. Too many have the misfortune of growing up in a place that lacks resources, so they don't have access to the high-quality medical care my own children now enjoy. Sometimes, the lack of access isn't because there are no nearby specialist doctors and hospitals. Sometimes, it's due to a lack of insurance coverage or an inability to pay for medical supplies and treatments. Often, families have overlapping problems, which are further exacerbated by bias and structural racism in health care—something you'll learn more about in this book.

Recently, we've learned that both pulse oximeters (monitors that measure the oxygen level in your blood) and medications for asthma can work differently in White people than in those who are darker skinned. This potentially life-saving information would have been discovered earlier if people of color had been included in research studies at a level commensurate with the disease burden they bear. I'm left wondering if, at least part of, the problem with controlling my asthma as a child was that too often, I was identified as being in distress too late and given treatments that were designed for someone else. You now understand I'm not being hyperbolic when I say I nearly died because of a lack of representation in clinical research. Hence, it's no coincidence that I now chair the board of an organization devoted to increasing diversity in clinical trials.

Racial disparities became painfully obvious during COVID-19, which hit communities of color harder than White communities. (You'll learn about the many reasons for that later.) The health status and opportunities of too many Americans have far more to do with zip codes—where you and the people like you live, learn, play, pray, and exist—than genetic codes. Under-resourced communities and individuals—Hispanics, Blacks, American Indians, Alaska Natives, those in rural populations, differently abled people, and members of the LGBTQ+ commu-nity to name but a few—are socially predisposed to have poorer health in America for a variety of reasons.

When I was appointed US surgeon general in 2017 and unanimously confirmed by the United States Senate, I was deter-mined to focus on public health—protecting and promoting the health and safety of families and communities across America. I was just as determined to promote health equity: ensuring every-one had the opportunity to be their healthiest self. I was eager to bring this up in any media exchange or public speaking I would do. The topic was and is personal to me. I know far too many people, family and friends, who suffer from high blood pressure, diabetes or prediabetes, and asthma. I can easily empathize with people who have the conditions I mentioned because I have all three myself and am on eight different medications to treat them.

Too often, politics complicated an already extremely diffi-cult situation of dealing with an unprecedented, once-in-a-cen-tury pandemic. This undoubtably made my work as the Nation's Doctor much harder. We need to clear away the BS and the bias that's dividing, confusing, and preventing us from achieving the health outcomes we want and are failing to achieve. Reflecting on how that happened, how that affected you and the people you care about, and what lessons can be learned will help us turn this ship around so that we no longer have to let politics stand in the way of our health.

Regardless of who is at the helm—who is president or which political party is in power—this ship, the wealthiest and most scientifically advanced on the planet, continually steers itself towards infectious disease icebergs. Why do we keep repeating the same mistakes; whether it's Bush and H1N1, Obama and Ebola, Trump (and Biden) with COVID-19, or Biden and mpox? Just as importantly, why can't we acknowledge that rearranging the deck chairs—or changing the captain—on the *Titanic* does nothing if we continually pursue the exact same course?

Despite the World Health Organization (WHO) saying COVID-19 no longer qualifies as a global emergency, and the Biden Administration ending US pandemic emergency declarations, many countries and communities have seen periodic surges in COVID-19–related hospitalizations and deaths—surges that haven't been contained even when travel restrictions are implemented. Not only are we not done with COVID-19, we also continue to see the flu and other infectious diseases like RSV (respiratory syncytial virus) affect too many Americans—often the most vulnerable of us—for several reasons.

First, we still don't have enough options for or availability of vaccines and treatments for current and emerging infectious diseases, including emerging variants of COVID-19. Second, we have high rates of mental health challenges, which further complicate physical health concerns. Mental health challenges intensified due to the stress and losses and economic pressures from the pandemic, and the volatile mood of the country, and we're still dealing with that fallout. Third, we'll continue to see infectious diseases harming us because we aren't adequately equipped, educated, or willing to protect ourselves as individuals or as a society. Shutting down schools and the economy, especially without clear and targeted outcome measures, can harm our health in many ways. However, not responding appropriately and aggressively, including shutting down when an infectious disease is overwhelming communities and hospitals, takes a huge toll on health and the future of our great nation—we've lost over one million Americans—including over 100,000 caregivers to COVID-19. The answer to how we can thrive economically while enjoying better health isn't to choose one over the other. Both are entangled in a complicated and messy way, and we must be willing to lean into that mess. The more that people are able to recognize and willing to set aside misinformation and disinformation, their biases, and their anger and fear, the better job we can all do in protecting ourselves from COVID-19, and whatever comes next.

To return to my *Titanic* metaphor, acknowledging that different people have different perspectives on what went wrong on the ship has been the source of multiple versions of the tale—and, consequently, different lessons learned. Some of those lessons have been about equity: rich people were far more likely to survive the *Titanic* than poor people. Some lessons were about the infrastructure and design of the ship, some were about hubris and how it can blind us to danger, and some were about safety protocols and crisis communication. A passenger on the ship will have a different perspective than a loved one (or member of the media) observing from the shore—especially if the passenger is in first class versus coach. The perspective of a someone who is public facing or "frontline"—a waiter or someone loading people onto lifeboats for instance—will differ from that of someone in the engine room or advising the captain at the helm. I served in all of those roles at various times while I was the surgeon general, so I have a both unique and comprehensive perspective on the situation. My goal isn't to convince you that I (or anyone else on the "ship") am without blame and couldn't have done things differently. My hope is that by sharing my perspective, I can convince you that many decisions, actions, and reactions may not have been as simple as they appeared from your vantage point.

I want to increase our understanding of the many complicated factors that lead us to continue charting a course towards that same iceberg—no matter how many times we've already hit it. My hope is that by sharing my version of this story, and by you reading it, we'll cause someone on the next journey to see beyond their limited view of the problem, and we'll be able to play a role in preventing another disaster. I believe this can happen despite our political divisiveness. I'm not giving up on our ability to come together—not yet.

I also will say upfront that I'd always prefer (and try) to leave politics out of the discussion. It's an obstacle to doing my job. I often tell this story to make my point: On the afternoon of May 15, 2018, I was on Delta flight 1827, scheduled to leave from Atlanta, Georgia, for Jackson, Mississippi. We'd not yet taxied onto the runway when the crew declared a medical emergency. A passenger had lost consciousness, and they asked if a doctor was aboard. Fortunately, I was there with two nurses, and we were able to respond, helping the man regain consciousness and escorting him to waiting medics. I did not first ask that man about his politics: Did he vote for Trump? Was he in favor of police reform?

Was he uncomfortable with people of color? And fortunately for me and that man, no one asked me to declare my loyalties or pass a political litmus test before they let me intervene as a physician. They didn't ask me to opine on how Trump or Biden would've chosen to handle the situation. All that mattered was whether I could assist in a crisis and perhaps help save a life. If any of those other questions were more important to me, I would not—and should not—be a doctor or public health policymaker.

Joining the Trump administration, I knew I would be steeped in politics for four years, regardless of my desire to remain politically neutral. I continue to believe that people's willingness to let themselves become caught up in the political drama cost us hundreds of thousands of lives. That frustration was a primary driver behind my choice to write this book. I don't care where you are on the political spectrum or whether you have no interest in politics whatsoever. We must remember that we're all Americans, and, in the words of Benjamin Franklin, "We either all hang together, or we shall all hang separately." We have to check our biases and recognize where they led us astray, or we'll all continue to hang our ability to protect ourselves.

In this book, I challenge you to recognize where you might have over- or underreacted, communicated ineffectively, or misunderstood others because you had a narrative (maybe planted by someone else) running through your head. Perhaps at times, you weren't willing or able to listen carefully, especially to objective health advice. We're all human, but getting stuck in anger, judgment, and blame will not prevent another pandemic or another life lost. We can't force other people to change, but we can change ourselves and make different choices going forward.

Choices that contribute to greater health and well-being in our homes, communities, and nation. Choices that are necessary if we are to avoid hitting that iceberg again.

• CHAPTER 1 •

NOT A SURGEON OR A GENERAL, BUT THE US SURGEON GENERAL

MOST PEOPLE KNOW ABOUT THE US surgeon general because of the warning labels on packages of cigarettes and the sides of wine bottles, but if asked what the job entails, they would draw a blank. I can fill that in: created back in 1817, the position of top doctor in the land was intended to be filled by a physician who would be the country's leading spokesperson on, and advocate for, public health. Being surgeon general means being the operational head of the US Public Health Service (USPHS) Commissioned Corps. Since the 1800s, when the USPHS was known as the Marine Hospital Service, we've used naval rankings, and as US surgeon general, I was commissioned as a three-star admiral. In other words, surgeons general are admirals and not generals. And while they are doctors, they usually aren't surgeons. I'm an anesthesiologist (the first anesthesiologist surgeon general ever). I know—it's confusing.

Like many of the twenty confirmed surgeons general who have served this country (though unlike most over the last several decades), I came into the job with both formal training and a specific, professional background in public health—a discipline that views problems from a different perspective than that of most people with a traditional medical background. I served as health commissioner for the State of Indiana from 2014–2017, having been appointed by then-governor Mike Pence. But despite my attempts to be known and referred to as the "Nation's Doctor" and the leading spokesperson on public health, the media continues to define me not as the twentieth US surgeon general but as "Trump's surgeon general." This attachment to the person who appointed them, especially for negative or sensationalistic purposes, is something the media has subjected no other surgeon general to (the current surgeon general is almost always referred to by the media as the "U.S. surgeon general," and the fact that he was appointed by Joe Biden is rarely mentioned in headlines or articles). It is dehumanizing, especially as Black people have fought for most of this country's history to be defined by their own hard work and not by the White men whom they work for or "belong" to. It also indicates a politicizing of the office and health policy, which I tried my best to avoid, and has serious consequences for all of us. The need to recognize and address this politicization, especially when we are perpetuating or falling victim to it, is one of the core lessons of the COVID-19 pandemic that inspired me to write this book.

As a child and even as a young medical student, I could not have foreseen becoming US surgeon general. My parents, schoolteachers from rural, southern Maryland, were worried that their severely asthmatic son might not live to adulthood at all—and certainly didn't consider I would one day end up in the White House as the second Black male to ever be confirmed as US surgeon general. And none of us could've further predicted

I'd be serving in what was arguably the most controversial presidential administration in all our lifetimes. But that's where I landed in 2017.

FIRST, YOU HAVE TO SEE IT

I grew up in the largely agricultural community of Mechanicsville, Maryland. My parents were educated and worked hard (my father served in the military and was the first in his family to get a college degree from the historically Black University of Maryland Eastern Shore), but we still often struggled to make ends meet. When I wasn't in the hospital due to my asthma, I was often outside working in the "fields," or the "woods," helping pick tobacco, load hay, or harvest firewood to make a few extra dollars. One of my worst asthma attacks ever—the one that caused me to be transported by helicopter to Washington, DC, for treatment—occurred after being exposed to allergens from working outside.

My parents were schoolteachers and taught their sons and daughter the value of the Catholic faith, doing well in school, an honest day's work, and respecting others—especially your elders. My family was close, both emotionally and geographically, as I literally lived within yelling distance of my grandparents, whose house was in front of ours, and my uncle and cousins, who lived next door. However, unlike my own kids today, I didn't grow up around doctors, lawyers, or even business owners. I had plenty of role models on how to be a good person and to work hard, but few to none who could advise me on pursuing a career that required an advanced degree.

I was an excellent student and in my school's gifted and talented program. I emphasize that because even after all I've accomplished, detractors will still attack my credentials, though in many ways, my training and professional experience made me far more qualified than even most doctors to serve as surgeon general. Detractors will also quickly resort to tired and racist accusations of affirmative action as the reason for my success. I graduated with a 3.94 GPA while in top-level and AP classes throughout my schooling. I was interested in science and math, and I'd participated in summer enrichment programs focused on engineering, so I had a clear sense of what I wanted to study at college. I was fortunate to receive a prestigious Meyerhoff scholarship (which serves as a pipeline for new PhDs and MDs) to attend the University of Maryland, Baltimore County, and to be mentored by the renowned Dr. Freeman Hrabowski.

Thanks to opportunities that came my way via the Meyerhoff Scholars Program, I had some formative internships that included working in the lab of a Nobel Prize–winner, studying hypertension in Zimbabwe, and spending a summer researching reactive airway disease in the Netherlands. During the latter, I worked with an MD, PhD, who was the first to expose me to what life was like as a physician.

I was intrigued, but it still didn't occur to me that I could have a job like his. He was White and from Europe. I was Black and from farmland USA. And regardless of seeing Bill Cosby play a physician on *The Cosby Show*, I didn't believe that people like me could be physicians. It may sound irrational, but for many young people, especially people of color, if you don't see it, it's hard to believe you can be it. Then, at a lecture in Baltimore that I attended through my scholarship program, I was able to hear Dr. Ben Carson, the famous Johns Hopkins neurosurgeon, speak. I sat there, gaping at him. Someone who looked like me was a *doctor?* I got to shake Dr. Carson's hand after his presentation, and I walked out of that auditorium with a new goal for my life. (Little could I have suspected at the time that Dr. Carson and I would both one day be the *only* black physicians advising our nation's leaders through a pandemic.)

I switched from engineering to biochemistry, knowing it would better prepare me for MCAT and medical school. Since I had also always been interested in learning what motivates people to behave in the ways they do, I started taking classes in psychology, eventually double majoring in psychology and biochemistry. Again, I finished with a 3.9 GPA, and that, along with my MCAT scores, earned me not only entrance to places like Harvard and Washington University in St. Louis, but also a full scholarship to Indiana University (IU), sponsored by the pharmaceutical company Eli Lilly. Through an accompanying summer internship at Eli Lilly during the summer before starting medical school, I met other Black medical doctors who would be mentors to me, and first learned about the difficulties companies like Eli Lilly faced in recruiting minorities to participate in clinical trials. I also learned about the many steps (and decades) it takes to get a drug from the idea stage to a thumbs up from the FDA. You see, even back then, I feel God was giving me opportunities to gain important perspectives (ones that would turn out to serve me well during a once-in-a-century pandemic).

While at IU, I became involved in professional societies like the American Medical Association, the Indiana State Medical

Association, and the Indiana Society of Anesthesiologists. I was also elected to serve as vice president of my class's governing council. These roles allowed me to learn how to be a leader and an effective public speaker and had me meeting with legislators, including then-congressman Mike Pence. I came to see that through legislative and regulatory advocacy, you could help shape policies that influence how and whether people receive quality health care—or any health care at all. Though I loved research and had been contemplating pursing both and MD and a PhD, that's when I recognized that life in a lab wasn't what I was destined for.

I ended up getting a master's degree in public health at the University of California–Berkeley with a focus on chronic disease prevention and worked for the City of Berkeley Public Health Division, helping develop a city plan to address nutrition and physical activity in underserved Black and Brown communities in the Oakland, California, area. I considered going into primary care medicine but was facing what we in the African American community call "the Black tax." That's when we make decisions about careers not just because of personal preference, but because many of us don't have the privilege of wealth—intergenerational or otherwise—that so many others take for granted. You feel the pressure to make enough money to not only secure your own future but to support your entire family. My parents had modest salaries and both of my brothers to look out for. My older brother is disabled, and my younger brother, Phillip, has substance use disorder (SUD) and has been in and out of jail and prison. My sister is smarter than all of us, yet that hasn't prevented her from struggling as a single mother. My parents have faced challenges emotionally, physically, and financially because of our situation. I enjoyed my anesthesia training, but unlike many of my White colleagues who had relatives or family acquaintances who were anesthesiologists, I knew very little about the field when I picked it. What I knew was that anesthesiologists can make twice as much as some primary care doctors do. Such an income would allow me to help out my family back in Maryland (which I still do) and support a wife who could stay home with our kids if that's what she decided to do. (By this time, I had married Lacey, whom I met during my first semester at IU.)

I continued to be involved in professional organizations, including the American Society of Anesthesiologists, where I worked my way to becoming chair of the professional diversity committee. I was living proof that outreach to young students of color could lead to greater diversity within the medical community, and I was glad to have the chance to draw more students like me into a field that is still mostly White.

By the time Congressman Mike Pence became governor, I was such a known entity in advocacy circles that he chose me, despite my young age and youthful appearance, to be in his cabinet and run the Indiana State Department of Health. When Governor Mike Pence then became vice president of the United States, I suspected I might be considered for a high-level position in the administration, but even so, I was deeply humbled, honored, and surprised when the offer came to be only America's twentieth surgeon general ever. (Statistically speaking, it's easier to become president than the surgeon general since there have been twice as many presidents in the last 150 years as there have been confirmed US surgeons general.)

SO MUCH FOR GLAMOR

Lacey and many of my relatives had mixed feelings about my appointment. I understood. After Donald Trump said of the tiki-torch terrorists of Charlottesville that there were "very fine people on both sides," my parents' opinion of Trump (especially my mother's), which was never high, sunk to a new low. "How could you?" some of my family members and friends asked. "How could you work for...that man?" Stephanie, one of my best friends from college, strongly advised me against it. "It's going to ruin your career," said others. (Imagine for a second being asked to serve in what most consider the most prestigious role in your entire profession and being told it was going to ruin your career.)

Interestingly my parents, lifelong Democrats (as most African Americans are), had been, and remain, very fond of former governor and vice president Pence. They met him on a few occasions and came away from those experiences with a deep respect for him despite their political differences. For one thing, he was gracious toward them—something they had not always experienced when dealing with White men in positions of authority. Also, like my parents, who arc devout Catholics, Mike Pence and his wife have a strong Christian faith. Both Mike Pence and my parents came from rural communities, which further secured a bond with him (as I've always said, when and if you can put aside politics, you'll often find you share far more in common with someone than you have differences). Momma and Daddy were extremely excited about my being given the opportunity to run the Indiana State Department of Health, a role in which I was the second African American, or person of color, and first in twenty years to serve. They were grateful to then governor Pence for seeing my potential and treating me well. Becoming the state health commissioner was more than they could have hoped for, and the pinnacle of my success—or so they thought.

When I discussed my new job with my friends and family, I explained that I wanted to have a seat at the table to represent people like us, who are too often ignored by those in power. As I often say to audiences whenever someone asks me, "How could you work for that man?," my retort then and now remains, "In the Bible, God never put anyone in a position where they'd be comfortable, but where they could make a difference. So, when God gave me an opportunity only one other Black man in history has been offered, how could I *not?*" My loved ones understood, but their feelings both about Trump and for me were so strong that it was difficult for them emotionally to accept my decision. Again Stephanie said, "I'm just afraid for *you* and how those people will treat you." The irony is she was right to be worried about how I would be treated but wrong about which "people" would be the ones most inclined to mistreat me—more on that later.

A year after I joined the administration, my parents came to the White House to see me give a speech for Black History Month honoring Black veterans alongside the president and first lady. Speaking at this event was one of my proudest personal moments. I was allowed to invite my father, who served in the army, my Uncle Vincent, a Vietnam War veteran, and my Uncle James, a disabled veteran. To go from a humble, rural upbringing to being able to host and honor my family at the White House was something most people can't even dream of. I told them we could pose for a family photo with the president. Though my mother was cordial during that brief interaction, she could not bring herself to actually speak to the president or even smile as the shutter snapped. Even in a moment when she was so obviously proud of her son, she did not want to convey that she was in any way happy to be standing next to "that man." That family picture hangs in my office at home, and when I look at it, I feel an intermingling of pride, love, amazement, and sorrow. It was an event that would make any mother burst with pride—the child you raised being honored at the White House by the president! Yet my mother's joy was so tempered by her feelings for Donald Trump that she could barely suppress a scowl. The emotional complexity of that experience was predictive of, and echoed by, what I experienced from many others during those four years as a Trump-appointee. I must admit I am still processing it all to this day.

In that photograph, my face expresses my happiness, eagerness, and determination. I wasn't naïve. I had worked as the top doc in ultraconservative Indiana. In fact, based on my successes in Indiana—among them, promoting syringe service programs and naloxone and securing legislative funding to address disparities in infant mortality—I felt confident I could figure out how to navigate the politics and still do what I came to do. I trusted Mike Pence. I also trusted that others who had worked their way into a position in public service high enough to merit them a White House ID badge would genuinely care about making our country "great" for everyone, even if we might disagree at times on how best to get there. Fostering and promoting public health might not have been at the top of the Trump administration's agenda (but let's be honest—polls show it's almost never at the top of any administration's agenda). Still, we were all in this together, serving the American people. I believed that and had faith that others did too.

I moved to DC in September of 2017 without my family as my kids had already started school in Indiana when I was confirmed. My wife and I decided we'd try to do the long-haul commute thing, with me coming home on the weekends. I knew plenty of other DC families who had similar arrangements, and they made it work.

Dealing with this arrangement as the surgeon general, however, was uniquely hard for me. Many of my speaking responsibilities would be on the weekends. Also, my schedule was far from predictable, and last-minute plane tickets proved to be prohibitively expensive, especially for someone now making a public servant's salary.

Seeing my kids and Bella (our dog) had typically been my emotional reward after a long day at work. We couldn't afford to maintain two separate residences, so I was staying in a garage in Virginia at my friends Chris and Jen's house. They were gracious hosts and had fixed up the garage nicely, but living alone and preparing meals in a college-dorm-room-sized microwave with food stored in a mini fridge was not how I pictured my life as a forty-five-year-old physician, must less as the US surgeon general. To this day, people imagine I was living a glamorous life with a driver and an entourage and government perks galore. The reality of my public service was that, despite being a three-star admiral, I was living out of a suitcase, separated from my family, and surviving off of apples, bananas, and microwaved ramen noodles while often using Uber to get from place to place.

This vagabond life lasted through Christmas, but it was hard on me. I lost ten pounds, which doesn't sound like much, but I started at 5'11" and 175, so I now looked almost skeletal (so said my mother at any rate). The situation was even harder on my wife. Our daughter was seven, but our boys were thirteen and eleven—challenging ages for boys even with a father around and even harder for a mother to deal with alone. Lacey and I made the difficult decision to put our dream home in Indiana—the house our kids had grown up in—on the market and rent a place near DC. The challenges of finding an affordable place for a family of five plus a dog in a good school district in the DC area while your wife is in a different state could be a book (or HGTV show) on its own. Frankly, doing so while trying to learn the ropes as US surgeon general, helping to raise three kids (who are all livid at you for making them move across the country), and preparing your house in different state for showing and sale in a down market is an experience I've mostly tried to block out. But by the grace of God and the patience and fortitude of my wife, we found a place in northern Virginia. The rent was more than our mortgage in Indiana, and the house was far smaller, far older, and in the words of our kids, far "stinkier." But we were together again.

I had my own ideas for what issues I wanted to prioritize as the "Nation's Doctor." Among my most important goals were to promote chronic disease prevention and to address the mental health and the opioid epidemics. However, what many people don't realize about the role of US surgeon general is that as the operational head of the Public Health Service—a six thousand-person organization—you spend a *lot* of your time dealing with oversight, management, and HR issues. There were hirings, firings, promotions, payroll, and IT crises every day. Your government support staff is nowhere near the size industry standards would recommend for an organization that big, so a lot of decision-making that ordinarily shouldn't and wouldn't come to the "CEO," too often did. Add to that the fact that the Trump administration (and the Obama administration before it) didn't see the value of maintaining and supporting a uniformed Public Health Service Commissioned Corps. (Both Democrats and Republicans have continually tried to cut the Corps.) Literally after a few weeks on the job, I was asked to present a plan to significantly decrease the size of the Corps to help save the government and taxpayers' money. A good 60–70 percent of my time on any given day was spent not addressing national health issues but trying to manage and save the US Public Health Service.

I also dealt with the challenge of largely interim (and political) leadership. Tom Price—the first Department of Health and Human Services (HHS) secretary and one who would leave his role amidst a scandal about his use of a private jet instead of a commercial airline—was already in place. Dr. Brett Giroir was appointed to be the assistant secretary for health—a position as that sat above mine and controlled both my budget and staffing as surgeon general. However, the job was filled by an interim caretaker for six months while Dr. Giroir was waiting to be confirmed by the Senate. The "acting" appointees in HHS were all told not to spend any unnecessary money, allow any new hires, or make any big decisions until the new team was in place. In other words, I had a bare-bones staff, no budget, and both hands tied behind my back as I tried to stand up to a new office, learn a new role, address a deadly opioid epidemic (and responses to three category 5 hurricanes), save a two-hundred-year-old uniformed service, and oh, be the nation's top health spokesperson.

Many people think the surgeon general hangs out in the White House and regularly interacts with the president, but that's not true. Beyond an initial interview for the job held in Trump Tower in 2016 and the aforementioned Black History Month event, I didn't encounter the president prior to 2020 and the pandemic. Public health is rarely a concern of any president unless, and until, there's a crisis. Despite the belief of many that I could just "tell" Donald Trump to take a particular action or say (or not say) a particular thing, there were no lunches in the White House Mess, no invites to the Oval Office, and no moments when the leader of the free world popped his head into my office to ask my opinion about health policy. Further, the surgeon general actually sits several layers down in the HHS organizational chart, so you must secure permission from (and often compete with) others who sit above you in the quest for White House attention for your own priorities.

Again, it's important to understand that that's the norm in every administration. I had been warned of this by prior surgeons general under both political parties who reached out to advise me. Those in public health don't get a lot of appreciation or respect despite our important roles. It's up to us to sound alarms and remind people repeatedly about topics that are mostly are out of sight, out of mind for them. And ironically if we do our job well and actually prevent a problem, we end up being seen as the boy who cried "wolf," because the disaster we warned about didn't unfold.

Further, more people die from smoking or obesity each year than from COVID-19, but the media is reactive to new, shocking, and acutely scary health information, not standard health advice about chronic disease prevention or mental health. Most people are too busy with other life concerns to focus on their own health, so they don't have the bandwidth or the desire to focus on what public health officials or health experts in the media have to say about often abstract or future threats. It's easy to change the channel to find a "sexier" topic than the latest study on stroke prevention, why you should drink less and lay off the sweets, what to do to avoid contracting the flu this season, or why you're not putting on enough sunscreen. Offering the public health information about "unsexy" topics is vitally important, however. As I highlighted in a *Surgeon General's Advisory*,[1] more people died from uncontrolled blood pressure in 2020 than from COVID-19.

Also, no one likes to hear the bad news that there are disparities in health care and treatment. Black moms and babies are dying, and structural racism is to blame? It's depressing, and people can feel helpless about (or blamed for) such systemic problems. Still, the US surgeon general's bully pulpit is an incredibly powerful one, and I was determined to do my best to use it effectively.

My prior role as Indiana health commissioner (Jocelyn Elders and I were the only two surgeons general in history to have run state health departments previous to taking on the role of Nation's Doctor) meant I had more media experience coming into the job than most, yet I can't consider myself an expert in communications like, say, a publicist or a journalist. I knew about two of the more notorious surgeons general's communication efforts. Dr. C. Everett Koop (who actually *was* a surgeon) served under President Ronald Reagan in the 1980s and was known for mailing information to every US household about exactly how HIV—the virus that causes AIDS—was transmitted. Many found this scandalous. (Interestingly enough, he was able to do this with the assistance of Dr. Anthony Fauci, who was part of the US Public Health Service Commissioned Corps at the time.) Dr. Joycelyn Elders, who served under Bill Clinton in the early 1990s, was forced out of her position after she suggested it might be a good idea to teach children about masturbation in sex education classes. You see, I wasn't the first to face public backlash for my messaging as surgeon general, and I won't be the last. Even so, health promotion is largely about communication, so I didn't have the luxury of fearing political challenges and unfair consequences for my advocacy. Long-faded headlines aside, on the heels of my local and national success advancing the controversial idea of harm reduction while serving as Indiana health commissioner, I took over the official US surgeon general's Twitter and Facebook accounts and began posting regularly.

Some were critical of my social media presence, suggesting that it was beneath the dignity my position as three-star admiral, but the majority of Americans—even doctors—report getting most of their health information online. If I was going to influence health decisions, that's where I needed to be. Unfortunately, despite being expected to be a national spokesperson on health, I had no dedicated social media support. I was composing and posting 50 to 75 percent of my own social media content on a daily basis. My kids know more about social media than I do.

That fact, along with my plainspoken nature, and willingness and desire to engage with anyone who I felt wanted to talk about health matters, would be a recipe for trouble. But you make do with what you've got. (I continue to feel social media can be an important forum for "town hall" health discussions.)

Soon after starting my job, I decided to focus on addressing our national opioid overdose crisis, which was an epidemic that predated the pandemic. I learned that while it hadn't been done in over a decade, past surgeons general had issued "advisories" to call attention to issues of critical health importance. I convinced HHS leadership to let me put out an advisory calling on more people to carry naloxone—an opioid overdose reversal agent that can save a life. Having it on hand is like teaching people CPR. And, critical to my "bosses," putting out this advisory was free. All I had to do was work with CDC, NIH, and FDA experts to compose it and use my influence as US surgeon general to promote it. Just as importantly, addressing the opioid epidemic was (and is) a rare bipartisan issue. Democrats and Republicans alike were happy to support and have a surgeon general standing alongside them fighting a public health enemy that didn't care what political party you belonged to. (And if we're being honest, this epidemic, which had raged for quite a while, was getting attention now because White kids were dying from it.) The opioid crisis allowed me to stand alongside Steny Hoyer (the Democrats' number two in the House) and Dick Durbin (Democratic number two in the Senate)—two people who vehemently opposed to the Trump administration. Despite outreach and offers to visit their states with them, I never was able to work with Democratic Senate leader Chuck Schumer or House

Speaker Nancy Pelosi on this issue. People in these positions may feel they have bigger priorities than health matters or that they may have bigger targets on their back if seen to be working with the "enemy." Perhaps even before COVID-19, crossing the aisle to work on a health issue that was killing Americans was a bridge too far for those in the highest political leadership positions.

Still, my naloxone advisory is one of the accomplishments I'm most proud of from my three plus years as US surgeon general. The advisory correlated with a 400 percent increase in naloxone dispensing nationwide, meaning tens of thousands of lives may have been saved by it. It felt good to advocate for an issue that is very personal to me, because as I said, one of my brothers suffers from substance use disorder. I hadn't had much success—even as surgeon general—in altering his trajectory, but maybe I could do something from a policy perspective that could save his life. Despite the obstacles, my tenure was off to a good start, and I was proud to be the Nation's Doctor and effectively wield the influence that came with the job.

Throughout my career, I've learned that if you aren't at the table, you will likely find yourself and your priorities on the menu. You have to be present in the "room where it happens," not only to present relevant information but also to give it important context so that decision-makers understand its weight. Also (and often), it's not what gets advanced by being in the room, but what you stop from being done that matters most. People often see and identify actions you specifically took, but they don't recognize the harm you prevented when you were present to say, "Hey, that idea's a problem because..." or "Did you think about how this might play out in poor/Black/rural areas?"

Being able to remain in the room and preserve your influence means maintaining a good rapport with the power brokers. I was fortunate to have had a good rapport with Vice President Mike Pence and Second Lady Karen Pence, and throughout my tenure, my seat at the table was often via direct or indirect invite from the Pences. That said, simply having a seat at the table doesn't guarantee you'll get the outcome you would like, but if you aren't there, you are guaranteed not to be heard. You have to be willing to take some losses and, at times, accept a half a loaf (versus no loaf at all). No job is perfect or without guardrails, and my job as surgeon general was no exception, yet few jobs give you access to the top-decision makers on the planet.

I was glad that being the US surgeon general gave me the platform to do the very difficult work I love. As a psychology major with substantial experience in health advocacy, I'm very familiar with how difficult it can be to get people to change their minds when it comes to health policy issues and to individually or collectively adopt healthier habits and lifestyles. Affecting public health is a long-term project that requires faith and patience. As I always tell audiences, the key word in "public health" is "public"—you need the public's buy in, so I had to listen, have an open mind, build trust, and take advantage of opportunities to be heard.

Again, I felt reasonably confident about my ability to communicate effectively, especially based on my past experiences, but even after dealing with three historic hurricanes in my first few months in office, I had no idea that another devastating storm— of a very different type—was coming.

• CHAPTER 2 •

RUMBLINGS FROM AFAR

ON JANUARY 1, 2020, CHINESE officials closed the Huanan Wet Market in Wuhan, China, out of concern about an infectious disease outbreak that seemed to have originated there. Within days, the WHO was informed, and within a week, Chinese public health officials identified that a novel coronavirus was the culprit. The CDC announced on January 20 that their lab had confirmed the first case in the US.[2] It's essential to understand how rapidly this situation evolved and that our surveillance and response was very heavily dependent on information from other countries. We also have to remember what else was occurring in our country at that time.

The presidential election and Democratic primary race were already on people's minds, but the major political story consuming the media and Congress's attention was President Trump's impeachment. This had begun in December—at exactly the same time the strange pneumonia cases began appearing in China. The media was all over that historical political event, so the brewing health story in China did not get the airplay or congressional attention it could or should have. Because of politics and media obsession with all things Trump, we overlooked the first of what would be many missed opportunities that could have helped us mount a more prompt and effective response. Further, China's refusal to share information or allow us to send in a CDC team to investigate the outbreak was a significant obstacle to our response.

As the new virus was just starting its spread across the globe, I was coincidentally getting ready to take a trip to American Samoa to get a ground-level view of a terrible measles outbreak that was responsible for 5,700 new cases and 83 deaths. Vaccine hesitancy was a concern in the continental US as well. In 2019, I had taken trips to New York and Washington state in response to measles outbreaks caused by low vaccination rates. Was I concerned about the novel coronavirus I was increasingly hearing about? Yes, but I wasn't alarmed. Every year, we experience new strains of respiratory viruses, but they usually fizzle out with little fanfare. It's usually the same old viruses, like flu and measles, and the failure of people to get their shots to prevent those diseases that ends up fueling the most deadly and worrisome annual outbreaks.

To give you some essential temporal and global perspective, we had fought SARS in 2003 without the need to develop a vaccine. We had survived outbreaks of Zika and H1N1 (swine flu) that were predicted to have a far greater societal impact than they actually did, even as bad as they were. In short, they eventually burned themselves out. The foreshadowing legacy of the Ebola outbreak in the US in 2014 was that far more people were harmed from delayed or denied care for other medical issues due to fear of Ebola than actually died from it. In other words, Americans had heard public health officials cry "wolf" before, so few people were going to pay attention to the latest infectious disease outbreak halfway across the world. Besides, non-stop coverage of a historical impeachment trial was keeping both the people and their elected leaders distracted.

Thanks to global commerce and travel, it was inevitable that COVID-19 would arrive in the US. The reality was not if, but when. The first actual US COVID-19 patient lived in Washington state, but had recently traveled to Wuhan, China. There was uncertainty about the virus's origin, but we were hearing that it was most likely transmitted from an animal to a human via a wet market, where people sell and buy exotic animals to eat. (Notably, the public health community had warned of the dangers of infectious disease transmission via wet markets. But, in a story as old as time, human convenience and keeping the economy churning had continued to win out over public health prudence.) Though there are convincing studies that now strongly suggest the origin of the virus to be an incidental wet market transmission, I have to acknowledge it is possible that the virus originated in a lab, and that possibility would capture and still holds the attention of many. Given the secrecy of the Chinese government, if the virus did escape a lab, it is highly improbable we will ever be given that information. In short, it's my belief that we will never know for certain how the virus originated. China's not suddenly going to say, "Hey guys, we want to come clean." But I personally believe the evidence suggesting it came from a wet market is the most compelling and likely to be correct.[3]

To me, what we can't afford to ignore isn't where the virus originated but how it is transmitted. The lack of transparency from China regarding the degree and type of person-to-person spread—particularly asymptomatic spread—is what actually most hamstrung our ability to make appropriate policy recommendations that could have saved US lives. It is well-documented that the CDC repeatedly attempted to send a team to China to help with initial investigations, but China refused. China—and by extension the WHO, which is still unwilling to call out China's bad behavior early in the pandemic—compromised our response. We must ensure this doesn't happen in the future.

We eventually learned from information leaking out of China that the virus was spread not just animal-to-human but person-to-person. China did share the genetic sequence of the virus, which allowed researchers around the world to begin developing tests and start working on a vaccine. Our hope—again, not without years of precedent—was that this virus would run its course and burn itself out sooner rather than later. The hope in the meantime was that we'd learn enough about it to keep it reasonably contained and under control. Despite our theoretical models, pandemic plans, and a largely political desire to accuse various individuals of downplaying the threat, it was decades of real-world experience that had prepared America—and politicians of both parties—to expect that the virus running its course and burning out would be the most likely outcome. The bigger concern for most of the nation was Trump, and an upcoming election.

TRAVEL BANS

In response to rapidly emerging cases and, unfortunately, a more slowly emerging understanding of the virus, major US airlines would restrict travel to and from China. With COVID-19 having appeared in several countries by January 31, the WHO issued a global health emergency—the sixth in its history.[4]

President Trump would be accused of racism for banning travel from China at the end of January 2020,[5] but too many forget many airlines actually banned flights in and out of China before he did. Travel restrictions are a public health tool that has been used for centuries to respond to infectious disease threats. My major issue with them is that when dealing with an infectious disease in a world of global travel and commerce, issuing and enforcing travel bans is like playing whack-a-mole. People will find a way to get to where they want to go; they can fly from China to Russia or Europe and then to the US, so a ban doesn't stop them—it just slows and reroutes them. Travel bans can also be unduly discriminatory and harmful to certain populations when applied in a kneejerk and/or xenophobic manner.

In January, airports that had handled the most international flights from "high-risk" areas were doing screenings, which expanded to other airports as more public alarm was raised. But the data on such screenings, both during and before the pandemic, illustrate that they required significant effort. What's more, they increased traveler inconvenience (which was bad for the economy and for the politicians who must answer to angry voters) and ultimately yielded us little actual protection. In other words, the "juice" often doesn't justify the "squeeze." Airport screenings made people *feel* a little safer—"Hey, at least they're doing something"—and bought us a little time to ramp up testing and develop a response plan (more so because it slowed down and discouraged travel for everyone than because we were actually catching infected individuals with COVID-19), but they didn't do all that much to actually stop the spread.

It's best to think of infectious diseases the way we think of Amazon deliveries: even if one hasn't arrived on your doorstep today from another country, it's probably no more than twenty-four hours away. By all means, we should consider travel bans to reduce the flow from the spigot for a finite period as we are adding other interventions. But a critical lesson—one that we continue to ignore in regard to many health issues—is that the sink will still overflow if you don't deal with the root of the problem. We needed to know more about how the coronavirus was spread and how to protect people, and we needed to quickly manufacture and distribute tests (and design a testing strategy) while working on other response measures.

Although travel to and from China was restricted, viruses don't care where they originated, where they first entered a human body, or who gets infected with them. They don't care about your beliefs, politics, race, ethnicity, age, gender, or health status. They only care about surviving, reproducing, and mutating when necessary to accomplish those first two goals. You must know your enemy to effectively fight it. Unfortunately, when it came to COVID-19, we didn't have the necessary knowledge and data to inform our battle plans, and that cost us dearly. More than any lack of urgency on the part of health officials or the administration, it was the secrecy practiced by China early in the pandemic that cost us valuable time—and lives.

HOW SERIOUS IS THIS CORONAVIRUS?

In January 2020, I was still doing a lot of public engagements. And I was starting to get questions about this emerging virus from China, while speaking to audiences and reporters about other health-related topics. Needing to know more about what was happening, so I could do my job as the Nation's Doctor, I pushed to be let into internal briefings about the virus—or at least to have access to the materials and readouts. Many are surprised to learn that early on, I wasn't invited to participate in HHS COVID-19 meetings. How could we go to war with a novel coronavirus without the "general" in the war room? But the problem was, despite my extensive public health background and experience managing outbreaks, I was seen as just a spokesperson and not someone who needed to be involved in strategy or operations discussions. Concerns about COVID-19 were increasing by the hour, but I was left to get most of my information the same way the rest of America did—by watching for updates in a media environment consumed by the impeachment proceedings.

When an infectious disease outbreak first occurs, you're prone to convince yourself you have matters under control. Not being in that position is frightening and dangerous, and the leaders of all countries naturally want to be seen as strong and capable, both by their own citizens and the rest of the world. Avoiding panic, even in a true crisis, is essential to maintaining order and stability. China's slow response to the danger of COVID-19 can be understood in these contexts. However, when you see that a respiratory virus is behaving quite differently from past viruses, including being both more transmissible and more deadly than past iterations, you have an obligation to share that information with the world. China's data, we would learn later, showed an extraordinary amount of spread—not just by confirmed cases in people who developed symptoms but also by asymptomatic individuals who tested positive. Though historically most seasonal respiratory viruses were thought to be primarily spread by large droplets or by fomites (any inanimate object that has become contaminated by a virus) that enter the human body when someone touches their nose or mouth, many around the world suspected this new virus was demonstrating characteristics of "airborne" transmission—despite what the WHO and the CDC were reporting. When you observe exponential increases in person-to-person transmission, your eyebrows *should* raise. The limited information from China early on was preventing public health officials from seeing (and believing) that SARS–CoV-2 wasn't behaving like the seasonal flu or its many cousins who seem to pop up and fizzle out from year to year.

"Airborne" can be a confusing term, so let me explain what it means when we talk about viruses. Most coronaviruses, including the one that causes the common cold, are significantly spread through droplets that are exhaled or expelled (for example, through a cough or a sneeze) into the air but quickly fall to the ground or onto nearby surfaces. Although the infected individual exhales the virus, it is thought to be largely contained within these droplets. In contrast, airborne viruses are not confined to droplets and are spread in particles that are smaller, lighter, and more diffuse. Since they don't fall as quickly as droplets do, airborne viruses can both travel further, even when not propelled by the force of a cough or sneeze, and pose a threat to others for much longer. Measles, for example, can exist for up to two hours in the airspace *after* an infected person leaves a room. Worse, if an airborne virus doesn't make itself known by causing obvious symptoms when one is infected (that is, the infection is "asymptomatic"), a person is likely to be unaware they are contagious, and therefore a threat to others.

The distinction between both airborne and non-airborne viruses and symptomatic and asymptomatic (or pre-symptomatic—the time before one shows symptoms, but is just beginning to be contagious) infections is nuanced but important. Throughout history, most all coronaviruses were widely thought by the scientific community to be transmitted by droplets *and* via people who were symptomatic. In other words, we could know even without a test that someone was sick, and we could largely protect ourselves by avoiding their droplets. We had no compelling reasons (or data from China) early on to expect this 2019 iteration of coronavirus would behave differently. Early 2020 advice from WHO, the CDC, and me, the surgeon general, was based on all we believed we knew up to that point about coronaviruses in general as well as what we knew at the time about *this* coronavirus.

For a virus spread by droplets and fomites (like the flu), we've always advised following the three C's:

Clean (your hands, washing them frequently)
Cover (your mouth and nose whenever coughing or sneezing)
Contain (stay home if you're sick)

Through social media, media interviews, and in-person meetings with people, I talked about the three C's and explained proper handwashing. I—and every other surgeon general in our lifetimes—gave out this advice every flu season, and America has come to expect it from us. We learned about handwashing as children, but unfortunately many people still don't know how to do it correctly to ensure that they are not transmitting germs, hence the need for regular reminders. (The CDC recommends to "scrub your hands for at least 20 seconds. Need a timer? Hum the 'Happy Birthday' song from beginning to end twice."[6]) I urged people to protect themselves from COVID-19, as well as from other respiratory infections (because we were in the thick of flu and RSV season) by practicing good hygiene. I advised them to cover coughs and sneezes and to avoid work or school if sick. I knew staying home when ill is difficult for many. Sick leave policies at many workplaces leave much to be desired. Even so, it was important for people to hear the message.

In late January, Dr. Anthony "Tony" Fauci, director of the National Institute of Allergy and Infectious Diseases, had just been appointed to the White House Coronavirus Task Force when he appeared on NBC to inform the general public about what we did and didn't know regarding COVID-19. He explained that we had five cases in the US and all were travel-related, but now we believed COVID-19 could be spread person-to-person and asymptomatically—though we still didn't know to what extent.

When asked about masks on *60 Minutes* in March, he said that "right now in the United States, people should not be walking around with masks" and "when you're in the middle of an outbreak, wearing a mask might make people feel a little bit better. And it might even block a droplet, but it's not providing the perfect protection that people think that it is. And often, there are unintended consequences. People keep fiddling with the mask and they keep touching their face."[7] Dr. Fauci's observation made sense: a small study of medical students at the University of New South Wales in Australia showed their unconscious face-fiddling occurred as often as twenty-three times an hour![8] If young medical professionals couldn't be expected to wear masks properly, it didn't seem prudent to advise the general public to do so—again especially because the scientific community *still* believed fomite transmission was a bigger and more preventable risk than airborne.

I publicly repeated this concern about masking based on the limited science we had available on the subject and on Dr. Fauci's statements. What he said made sense (again, based on a presumption of primarily droplet and fomite transmission). And after all, Dr. Fauci had been studying infectious diseases for fifty years and was among the most highly respected individuals in the virology and public health community, even before the pandemic.

The available data suggested most Americans were still seemingly at low-risk for infection, but as Dr. Fauci emphasized, the situation was ever evolving. At this point, we knew that people with underlying conditions would be at a higher risk for hospitalization and death (as is the case with the flu), but we did not know how high asymptomatic spread was, or how badly this virus was going to impact certain communities. Without widespread testing and reporting, there was no real way to know how contagious or deadly the virus was. And we did not realize the extent to which it was airborne.

WE ONLY KNEW WHAT WE KNEW

To give you some perspective, the CDC didn't declare COVID-19 to be airborne until May 2021,[9] and the WHO didn't do so until December 2021.[10] You read that right. Despite their best intentions, the task force and the administration were bound to make at least some mistakes in early 2020, because our understanding of SARS–CoV-2 was minimal and it was framed through the lens of our experience with past coronaviruses. The lack of transparency from China was crippling—remember we lacked adequate testing or surveillance capabilities of our own—and in terms of the data that *was* available, the CDC has a culture of methodical analysis (some say overanalysis). It didn't have the infrastructure or authority to quickly respond to our need for good, representative data from states regarding COVID-19 infections. It may seem unbelievable, but initially, all COVID-19 tests had to be approved by and then sent to the CDC. So, while many suspected the virus was more contagious than it first appeared, the task force and I were in the difficult position of needing to make hugely consequential national policy recommendations without the data to confirm those suspicions. I like to say we were driving the car down the road at night, without headlights, and turning the wheel only after we hit something.

Had the task force or the CDC made a declaration about the airborne nature of the virus only to have to reverse themselves if data later showed them to be wrong, public trust would have eroded. Ironically, public trust was eroded anyway, because they made the declaration too late. I often talk about Colin Powell, who advised and mentored me during the pandemic, and his famous 40/70 rule: you won't get every decision or judgment right, but if you act before you have 40 percent of the information on a topic at hand, you'll significantly increase your likelihood of being wrong. However, if you delay decision-making much beyond having 70 percent of the necessary information, any action will have far less influence and impact. Aim for making that decision or judgment when you have between 40 and 70 percent to get the best results. It's challenging to wait for information when faced with the threat of people suffering and dying. And it's challenging to act quickly when you're the CDC, which is designed to be slow and deliberative and whom people will attack, even if they are wrong only 1 percent of the time. Preventing all harm would have been impossible, but I wish we'd had a response system that allowed us to more easily follow the 40/70 rule. We should have done better, and I want to talk frankly about what happened and why so it doesn't happen again.

The troubling news is that we have already seen many of the same mistakes from our flawed COVID-19 response with the 2022 mpox (formerly known as monkeypox) outbreak— for example, not getting tests or vaccines or treatments to the people at highest risk quickly enough. With COVID-19, we needed to ramp up testing and ensure that the distribution of tests made sense and that there were minimal delays in getting or responding to results. We relied on the CDC, whose structure was set up more to deliver long considered advice than to launch an emergency response. And when it actually is responding, the CDC is more accustomed to dealing with smaller regional health emergencies (such as an outbreak of measles in New York) than widespread national ones. Worse, despite talk of "defunding" the CDC, from a resource perspective, it is woefully outdated and underfunded (more on that later) to manage the critical tasks at hand. Unlike with other governmental entities, speed is neither core to their culture, nor facilitated by their funding, resources, and authorities. I saw for myself the big shift that occurred when the White House Task Force began to involve ASPR, FEMA, and the military. It was like the Flash showed up.

We couldn't know how infectious COVID-19 was until we had mass testing. Unfortunately, we've never at any point in the pandemic had a true national testing strategy, and it took us years to better track the appearance and characteristics of new variants, which is why we always seem to be playing catch up with this perpetually evolving coronavirus. Still, ethically and practically, the early focus needed to be on the most vulnerable—those most likely to be hospitalized or to die from COVID-19—and on those caring for them. I actually fell into both high-risk categories due to having asthma and being a practicing physician. In early 2020, I was still performing anesthesia cases at Walter Reed Hospital (to my knowledge, I was the only US surgeon general in modern times to continue regularly practicing medicine while in office). I had to push for special permission (from the HHS Secretary) to continue working, just as I had back in Indiana when I was state health commissioner. I wanted to maintain my clinical credibility by staying connected to the practice of medicine, and I also wanted to have day-to-day insights into how policies we crafted were playing out on the ground level. That choice to stay connected to the "boots on the ground" would later give me critical information—information that contradicted much of what politicians and policymakers, even those on the COVID-19 task force, would say about how well states and institutions were faring with this once-in-century health crisis.

GIVE ME A SEAT ALREADY!

Throughout February, whenever I talked to the press, reporters would inevitably bring up the new coronavirus—a topic I wasn't being briefed on and wasn't cleared to speak on. I was the US surgeon general, though, so whether I was there to talk about the opioid epidemic, maternal mortality, or high blood pressure, any health questions were fair game when the cameras started rolling. The rumbling from China was becoming a roar, and the questions I was getting made me increasingly uncomfortable. I continued to work on other important health issues including the first surgeon general's report on smoking cessation in thirty years, which I released in January of 2020. But I also began pushing even harder to attend the internal COVID-19 briefings. As the Nation's Doctor, I didn't want to be out there winging it.

On one of my last "non COVID" trips, I flew to New Orleans to present at a national conference on smoking. While there, I visited a local community health center where they had instituted some of the earliest COVID-19 testing, for vulnerable HIV-positive patients. I stopped at a local academic medical center and heard prescient concerns about bed capacity if the situation worsened—an understandable fear given that Mardi Gras was looming. I walked outside my hotel and down Bourbon Street, and while alcohol has a way of alleviating anxiety about interacting with strangers, I noticed people were keeping their distance from one another more than in the past. Concern was increasing that COVID-19 might not fizzle out like Ebola, Zika, or H1N1 had. Maybe this particular virus would be the one we all feared, despite our recent successes containing other infectious diseases. I wanted to know more and be a part of the strategizing, but at the time, I was relegated to the road—where, ironically, I was getting better ground-level intel than those running the response back in DC. Though the administration was still being told (and felt) that we had sufficient testing on a national level to meet current needs, working medical professionals were telling me they were woefully short of testing capabilities sufficient to adequately identify and control local spread.

As I waited for my return flight from DC to take off from New Orleans, I wanted to both calm fears and give people practical advice. I tweeted a video of myself on the airplane telling people that currently, I was still more concerned about the flu than the coronavirus. I did this because panic—and panic buying—was beginning to surge, and because even at that point, it truly was what the available data was telling us. Documented flu cases *far* outstripped known COVID-19 cases in the US at that time, and frankly, at that point I personally felt more concerned about the flu for my own family and myself than I did about COVID-19. By that point in time, we'd recorded 149 pediatric flu deaths vs 41 covid deaths (which were almost entirely in the elderly or immune compromised). In fact, the CDC flu report from that week stated hospitalization rates for flu in children 0-4 and adults 18-49 "are now the highest CDC has on record for these age groups, surpassing the rate reported during the 2009 H1N1 pandemic." The word from China and the CDC, however, was that we were gaining a foothold in our understanding of the virus and that we had, or would quickly have, sufficient tools to deal with this new threat. In my video, I urged everyone to get vaccinated for the flu and to follow the three C's. I also felt that since most all health experts and organizations were still saying SARS–CoV-2 was likely to behave similarly to past respiratory viruses, protecting oneself from the flu would have the secondary benefit of protecting oneself from COVID-19. I was on the wrong (and low) side of Colin Powell's 40/70 rule, only I didn't know it.

By now, Italy had quarantined fifty thousand people and cancelled several public events.[11] Dozens of countries, including ours, were limiting travel to and from China.[12] President Trump decided that we needed a stronger, more formal, and government-wide response, and in late February, I was asked to join the White House Coronavirus Task Force, by Vice President Pence. Finally, I was finally in the war room and determined to build the necessary relationships with other Task Force members that would lead to the best possible outcomes—or so I thought.

• CHAPTER 3 •

IN THE WAR ROOM

EVERY YEAR, INFECTIOUS DISEASE OUTBREAKS emerge across the globe—whether it's bird flu, mpox, or a flare-up of Ebola. In response, HHS typically assembles a response team with people from the CDC, the ASPR (Administration for Strategic Preparedness and Response), NIH, FDA, and other relevant agencies to develop policies to prevent spread. The original White House Coronavirus Task Force reported mainly to an audience of one: HHS secretary Alex Azar. (It's worth noting that due to the demographic makeup of those in leadership, these meetings—in most all administrations—often include no one who represents, or can speak to, the concerns of underrepresented minorities, even though those very groups often bear the brunt of harm when a new infectious disease spreads.) As the COVID-19 situation increased in magnitude so did the policy implications, meaning the nature of the task force had to evolve. We needed more than just CDC input, and we needed to talk about more than health policy. We needed a room full of experts weighing in on the impact of the disease, not just on hospitals and doctors' offices but on American life—agriculture, transportation, immigration, and housing. That meant gathering secretaries and policymakers from various cabinet agencies in the "war room."

In late February, the president appointed vice president Mike Pence to chair the COVID-19 task force. This new and larger task force would meet daily and with other experts when new problems inevitably arose. For the aforementioned reasons, several new members were added (and some were removed). At this point, the vice president recommended I be added to the list, and I was.

To keep people safe and stop the spread of a highly contagious and deadly disease, one has to consider a wide variety of community living situations, habits, and cultures, among other factors. America's diversity is a great asset, but it also can pose tremendous challenges, as anyone in public health knows. We needed a task force that could speak to the myriad problems that might arise in different communities and sectors from varying policy decisions. In summarizing who was on the task force and how they contributed, I hope to make the case that, in times of crisis, a variety of voices in the war room is essential (and I know that my presence alone increased the diversity in the room in a very tangible and visible way).

Some might argue that the presence of Steve Mnuchin, the secretary of the Treasury, on the task force represented a callous emphasis on the economic effects of COVID-19. However, in my opinion, his presence was crucial. While surgeon general, I prepared a first-of-its-kind report on health and the economy that pointed out something I often share with people who are prone to focus on health at the exclusion of finance and business or vice versa: health crises impact finances, which in turn impact health. You can see this at the micro-level with a family. If one member develops cancer or has a serious accident, they might lose their job. The emotional and financial stress on everyone in the family might cause the person or their spouse to become anxious or depressed. They might begin to self-medicate with alcohol or other substances—or both. The family may not have insurance, or their insurance may be inadequate, forcing a choice between paying for medical care and paying the rent. (Medical expenses are one of the leading causes of bankruptcy in the US as people struggle to pay for food and housing along with medical bills.) The financial stress on a couple can lead to divorce, domestic violence, or even suicide. Even if family members are able to continue working, they are more prone to absences and being less attentive and productive while on the job. Multiply that scenario by millions and then consider that the leading causes of disease and death in the US—cancer, heart disease, and now COVID-19—are often preventable. In the case of COVID-19, there could have been significant consequences for our nation's health if schools and businesses didn't shut down—at least for a while—but there were also workforce consequences when they did: many parents had to stay home from work to care for children who were no longer in school. You can't separate economics from health.

Another new task force attendee was secretary of agriculture Sonny Perdue. It's hard to forget the state of grocery stores in the spring of 2020—the cold and flu medicine aisles were stripped bare, toilet paper was being hoarded, and store shelves had no meat. Secretary Perdue was able to give us insight into the mystery of the latter. Unlike with toilet paper and cold medicine shortages, the issue wasn't panic buying and hoarding. The meat shortage pointed to a population that was becoming infected in disproportionately high numbers: Hispanics and Latinos, particularly first-generation immigrants and those in close contact with them. Both legal and illegal immigrants to this country, many of whom come from Mexico, Central America, and South America, are over-represented in the food processing industry where language barriers and immigration status are not as problematic as they are in other jobs. Low-income immigrants are likely to live in suboptimal housing (often makeshift shacks). They typically get no paid time off and have little savings to provide a cushion if their paychecks are docked when they take a sick day. If infected, they're unlikely to be able to isolate in a place where there's little risk of infecting others. If they or their family members are in the US illegally, the fear of deportation often prevents them from seeking medical attention.

Secretary Perdue pointed to the many outbreaks in meat processing plants. The problem was so severe that pigs were being exterminated and their carcasses burned because there weren't enough workers to process the meat. That agricultural consequence alerted many in the task force and government to the urgency of addressing the COVID-19 burden in Hispanic and Latino communities. It also forced us to reckon with the real-world implications of strict and prolonged quarantine policies for those who may have been exposed. We discussed that we would see more outbreaks if we didn't do three things: 1) provide sufficient guidance to these communities; 2) make resources such as testing and PPE easily accessible; and 3) remove the fear of deportation or inability to become a permanent US citizen if immigrants went to emergency rooms. The meatpacking facility outbreaks would affect our ability to both "flatten the curve" and feed our society at a time of supply chain interruption.

What role could the Department of Transportation (DOT) play? If you keep in mind that you can't treat the economy and public health as existing on their own policy-planets, the task force needed DOT's input on what was happening not just with airlines but also with buses, trains, cruise ships, and so on. We needed to understand and weigh the danger of strangers congregating in tight spaces against the harm to our country if we overly constrained travel. We weren't just concerned about businesses being interrupted due to travel restrictions. We needed pandemic responders to be able to travel to new hotspots, and organ transplants to get from state to state. Airlines use HEPA filters to clean the cabin air, so flight attendants, pilots, and passengers were at lower risk than people on trains and buses, but that brings up another point. As a society, we tend to render service workers invisible. We are so focused on what we're doing and where we are going that we don't pay much mind to the bus driver, the TSA agent, or the grocery worker, yet all of these people, and more, are at elevated risk for contracting COVID-19 simply by making our lives more convenient. Just try to estimate the number of people you encounter when traveling. Also, we knew that travel would pick up as spring break and Easter approached, and summer travel would soon follow. We had to consider how to make it safer and if and when to stop it all together.

Fittingly, we also had military officials in the war room. They partnered with DOT and HHS to address one of the biggest challenges of the pandemic, one that also turned out to be one of the biggest and least spoken of successes in my opinion: the handling of incoming cruise ship passengers. Cruise ships congregate thousands of people from all over the world in extremely close quarters. Additionally, many of the guests are older; the average age on the cruise ships in question was well over sixty, correlating with the age of high-risk for hospitalization from COVID-19. States began refusing to let cruise ships with onboard outbreaks disembark. I was fielding frantic calls from friends and colleagues with family members stuck on cruise ships asking if I could help. Assistant secretary of ASPR Robert Kadlec was charged with orchestrating evacuations. Exposed passengers had to quarantine for fourteen days even if they initially tested negative (we set them up on military bases). All needed to eventually travel home safely, often crossing several state lines to do so. First, we had to acutely deal with the potential disaster of thousands of incoming passengers disembarking and dispersing across the country while possibly carrying and spreading a deadly virus. Then we had to ask ourselves, should we recommend that no new cruises be allowed to leave, and what effect would such a decision have on the economies and the health of port cities in states such as Florida, Texas, and California? We don't hear or talk much about the cruise ships as we discuss the pandemic, but they were a disaster waiting to happen—a disaster that was fortunately averted.

Homeland Security was another essential part of the task force. They help manage the unfathomably large number of people who cross into and out of the US every day—not just illegal but legal crossings involving our land borders with Mexico and Canada. (We focus on the southern border but you can't, or at least shouldn't, treat people coming into the US over one border differently from those crossing another.) By some estimates, over a million people cross our borders every day—to buy goods, visit family, obtain medical care, or work if their job is on one side of the border and their home on the other. Governors of border states often talk tough about and focus on illegal immigration, but they know that people who cross the border are a crucial part of their state's economies, contributing through the work they do and the money they spend. Chad Wolf had taken on the role of secretary of Homeland Security in November 2019 and was serving in an "acting" capacity without full authorities or flexibilities. Still, he offered critical insights when discussing the effect of pandemic policy on our ability to keep our country safe and our economy functioning. Well into the Biden administration, officials were still grappling with tough choices about if and when to end Title 42 (the pandemic border policy used to expel immigrants for the sake of national public health).

The CDC was receiving incomplete data and passing it on to the task force. They were constantly promising to do better but were mostly unable to deliver. The task force would have regular calls with governors, most of whom insisted that they had matters under control in their state, whether or not that was completely true. No one wanted to be the governor or state "in trouble." Meanwhile, because of the relationships I'd fostered over the years with state health commissioners, I was receiving texts and calls telling me the ground truth about their difficulties procuring PPE and tests and getting them to those who most needed them. Simultaneously, Dr. Fauci and I were hearing from our physician colleagues on the ground that no, they were not getting the resources they needed to do their jobs and stay safe. I've said that I believe representation matters, but the experiences of the White House Coronavirus Task Force proved that in ways you might not expect.

As I reflect back on the early days of the task force, at least two people should have had a bigger and sooner presence: Seema Verma, head of the Centers for Medicare and Medicaid Services (CMS), and secretary of education Betsy DeVos. Given the lack of demographic diversity on the task force, Administrator Verma's input and insights as a mother and person of color were helpful (as were my own personal experiences as a father of school-age kids and Black man). However, she proved to be a crucial team member for another reason: she was in charge of the eight-hundred-pound gorilla of US healthcare funding, the Centers for Medicare and Medicaid Services (CMS). I often say we don't have a health care system in this country so much as we have a sickness reimbursement system, and CMS determines the rules and rates paid to treat those sicknesses and gets the checks in the mail. Administrator Verma could (and after being added to the task force by Vice President Pence, did) provide carrots to incentivize hospital- and nursing home–reporting and policy changes. And she could withhold reimbursements if entities did not give us the data we were asking for—a "stick" that often proved more influential than any carrot we dangled before them. After she became involved, the flow of data from hospitals improved dramatically. I was reminded that if you don't have the person who is paying the bills sitting at the table, you won't be able to push the buttons that make vital functions of the US healthcare machine run or change the behaviors of those pulling the machine's levers.

I said earlier in this book that we need to openly acknowledge faults in our response so we can do better next time. Not having an earlier and stronger contribution from Secretary DeVos's department of education was a critical mistake. We had no clue how much difficulty schools would have setting up virtual learning, especially in rural and under-resourced urban communities. And just as we had a myriad of blind spots regarding health data, we had no visibility into the impact that missed school was having on our youth.

WHAT WERE WE OVERLOOKING?

From my perspective, it was very forward-thinking of the administration to have Housing and Urban Development secretary Dr. Ben Carson on the task force. First, it was nice to have another physician—particularly an African American male—on the task force to join me. (It's noteworthy that I can't name a single African American physician, must less a Black male, involved with the current administration's COVID-19 response or messaging. And Black male doctors play a special role in improving health outcomes for Black men who have worse health and less longevity than women and men of other races.) I believe Secretary Carson was invited mostly because of his stature in the administration and his influence with the president, as opposed to an inherent recognition that housing would be an important part of the pandemic response. Still, he was a valuable addition to the team, because like me, he grew up in a low-income family, which gave him a perspective many in the room didn't have. When you know what it's like to live in a family that operates from paycheck to paycheck, you tend to remember folks who don't have a fully furnished basement to quarantine in or a job they can do remotely. Secretary Carson and I pointed out early on that if we were going to tell people to stay home, we needed to give them the support and resources to do so.

Agency representation mattered, but so did the fact that several people (though not enough) came to the table with perspectives shaped by experiences that those in the White House who were older, White, and male didn't have. The only woman regularly seated at the table was a grandmother, Dr. Deborah "Deb" Birx. I think she had an easier time recognizing that a lack of childcare would create a considerable burden on families and, in particular, women than the men did. Even so, rarely was there someone in the room who was trying to do their job, in person or remotely, while simultaneously trying to ensure that their kids were out of bed, logged onto their classes on time, paying attention, and actually learning something at home. My wife, Lacey, was sharing with me her challenges of getting our three kids to stay focused on their school lessons, so I brought up some of her experiences as a pandemic mom. When you're at the table, you also have to think of who is not in the room, and the perspective of moms was often absent. (In fact, while I interacted with Ivanka Trump and Kellyanne Conway, politics was rarely, if ever, the focus of our conversations. I knew them and related to them as parents concerned about their kids at this stressful time. Seeing them, I was reminded of how many women were struggling to balance family life, their kids' schooling, and their careers.)

No one on the task force had babies or preschoolers and was stuck without daycare. We all had broadband access and laptops and were computer literate, but millions of Americans lacked these advantages. All of us had high-quality health insurance, while the rest of the country had a patchwork system and too many people had *no* insurance at all (yet another big issue we needed Administrator Verma's CMS influence to address). We had no direct input from the Native American population, whose people were isolated from many of the resources those of us on the task force took for granted. (I made it a point to visit reservations and speak to tribal leaders throughout the pandemic, but that's not the same as having real representation at the table.) Many on reservations not only lacked medical facilities and broadband for virtual schooling, but they also lacked running water.

We would also later realize that we gave short shrift to other pandemic-related problems that included a sudden lack of day-care for working parents, rising mental health crises and challenges, and increases in substance misuse and drug overdoses[13] and domestic violence.[14] Both the pandemic and our policies to respond to it were exacerbating these issues, and the political and social divisiveness that millions of Americans became swept up in affected people's emotional and physical resilience when they most needed it to be strong.

My impression was that, despite what you may have heard in the media or from politicians and others hostile to the Trump administration, everyone on the task force cared deeply about helping the American people conquer COVID-19. Everyone took the threat seriously. They just saw policy tradeoffs through different lenses. Those of us who were doctors were probably more aware than the others that the unfolding pandemic was exposing long-standing health inequities in our country. Still, it wasn't as if people on the task force were knowingly or willingly looking to let the virus spread and harm marginalized communities (at least, not in the beginning—but more on that later).

No one likes to discuss big, seemingly intractable problems. Even so, I rarely felt stifled when bringing up uncomfortable truths or pointing out that we needed to be aware of the special challenges certain groups faced—especially when Vice President Pence was running the meetings. The vice president had assured me he would always support me in doing my job and giving the public accurate health information. His promise is why I felt confident giving the facts about hydroxychloroquine (HQC), even going on one of the president's favorite shows and contradicting his enthusiasm about HQC in an early 2020 interview with Sean Hannity. (Hannity abruptly ended the interview when it became apparent that I wasn't going to be a full-throated supporter of HQC for all.)[15] I caught no flak for it from the White House because I stuck to the known science and avoided commenting on the president or his remarks—positively or negatively. (People are fond of saying that I should have made it a priority to criticize the president each and every time he said something that the scientific community didn't agree with—but no matter the surgeon general or the administration, you won't be able to advocate for the issues you care about for long if you make a habit of publicly attacking your boss.)

I don't agree with everything Vice President Mike Pence has done or said about health matters. Heck, I don't agree with everything my dad or my wife believes or says. But in working closely with Vice President Pence on multiple health crises over the years, I've always known him to display a deliberative, calming, and inclusive leadership style. Just before each task force meeting adjourned, Vice President Pence would ask us doctors, "Is there anything you're not telling us that we need to know?" (Whenever the doctors felt there was a critical policy point the task force or president was missing or underappreciating, the strategy was to try to go through me to get the information to the vice president rather than to try to work through the White House staff who surrounded the president.)

As the meetings continued, I increasingly felt the burden of gathering insights from a wide variety of Americans about their challenges and sharing them with the task force. Could I represent all of them effectively? Was I on top of all of their various challenges? Trying to speak for all these constituencies while also offering my life experiences to shape and inform the conversations would become even more critical as both viral spread and panic heated up. It was all the more stressful because many of the same marginalized groups I was fighting for hated the president. As such, they missed no opportunity to criticize him and anyone associated with him (for example, yours truly)—especially as the election drew nearer.

In the meantime, I was wrestling with how to communicate our emerging and evolving knowledge about the virus and the risk of infection, hospitalization, and death to a scared and increasingly angry nation. I often did it on hostile and agenda-driven news shows and in interviews where my message was framed by someone else and my speaking time to explain nuanced information and policies was limited to two to three minutes. I had done plenty of public speaking on health before, but the hot seat would turn out to be much hotter than I (or anyone) had ever experienced.

• CHAPTER 4 •

IN THE MEDIA HOT SEAT

WHILE THE TASK FORCE WAS looking at the available data and constantly updating each other on what we knew, and what, if any, strategy changes we should consider, I never forgot the lives that were at stake, including the lives of vulnerable people I knew and cared deeply about. I needed the American people to trust me and was committed to transparency. We had to share and explain what we knew but also what we didn't know—and what we were doing to learn more.

Talking about unknowns is difficult when people want you to speak in soundbites and tweets. It's also tricky when the White House is managing—and at times limiting—whom you can speak to. At one point early on in my tenure, I had my hand smacked when I agreed to speak about the opioid epidemic to Lester Holt at NBC without clearing it—not because of what I said but because NBC was perceived as hostile to the administration.

The Trump administration wasn't the first to exert control over which reporters their appointees could talk to, hoping to avoid hostile and often unfair interviews and reporting. Politically, no White House wants to encourage the press to report on problems. They want to sell solutions and successes. Democratic appointees, including the Biden administration's public health officials, talk far less (or not at all) to Fox News and Newsmax, and Republican administrations are wary of MSNBC and CNN. I always made a point to try and talk to a "Left"-leaning media outlet if I had just talked to one that leaned "right." I kept in touch with former surgeons general, and when we compared notes, it actually seemed I was less constrained than they were.

Often, I faced the unenviable task of explaining to the public any guideline changes that would happen as our understanding of the virus, its clinical manifestations, and the patients who were affected by them evolved. The need for immediate guidance to help states and medical personnel meant we were building the policy plane as we were flying it. New information was coming in daily, and I was getting information second- or third-hand, often after the CDC had already publicly released (or leaked) guidance or reports without warning us. I found myself giving advice that some felt contradicted what I'd said just weeks or even days prior. Dr. Deb Birx was busy coordinating the health contributions of the task force and working with Dr. Robert Redfield of the CDC to get better data. Dr. Ben Carson had his hands full as the head of HUD and as a Cabinet Secretary of an administration revving up for a brutal election fight. I and Dr. Fauci would become the doctors primarily tasked with communicating to the public, which we did through traditional and social media.

Dr. Fauci is an infectious disease expert and researcher, and a retired admiral in the US public health service. He'd managed to fly under the general public's radar during most of his fifty years of public service. He has advised not only several presidents but also surgeons general. In early 2020, Dr. Fauci was constantly gathering info via his connections with NIH and the WHO to better understand what was going on, but he would also speak to the press. After all, he'd been doing that as early as the Reagan administration and our initial insights into HIV. I had press experience from my time as a state health commissioner, where I had to deal with messaging about an Indiana HIV outbreak that was the worst outbreak related to injection drug use in the history of the US. I also had several hundred thousand Twitter followers, which was a good resource for communication, but also represented a minefield of potential problems (more on that later). Given my bully pulpit, the task force and White House agreed that I had a unique role to play in getting information and guidance out, particularly to marginalized communities.

Dr. Fauci and I spent long days at the White House attending task force meetings before catching up on our "regular" jobs. Afterward, we would often meet over the phone to discuss what to say publicly on the following morning's news shows. In a sense, the two of us became the sacrificial lambs—the messengers who bore the brunt of the anger about the messages the task force was sending, or the contextual information we didn't have. If you didn't like the guidelines, if the changing scientific information angered you, we were the ones the public and the media threw darts at. I certainly didn't expect the blowback from that part of the job—simply giving updates to the public—to be quite as intense or as political framed and motivated as it turned out to be. I and many other public health officials received hateful emails, and I even received death threats delivered to my house. But what most flummoxed me was being attacked by the very groups I was most trying to help. Pre-pandemic (and pre-election year), people from those groups were happy to have me representing them and were supporters, often beseeching me to speak at their events. But I'd also never before had to communicate about a once-in-a-century virus—one occurring on the heels of an impeachment trial of one of the most polarizing individuals in history, and during a presidential election taking place in an atmosphere of once-in-a-generation racial acrimony and divisiveness. This historical context, unrelated to the actual science, shaped both our messages (for example, does social distancing mean people shouldn't vote in primary elections? Or attend George Floyd protests?) and how they were received. Even when Dr. Fauci (whom most of America would come to view as leaning Left) and I (whom most of America viewed as leaning right) were saying the exact same things, they were often framed and highlighted differently by the media and public.

SERIOUSLY, PEOPLE. STOP BUYING MASKS!

Dr. Fauci and I had been getting desperate calls and emails from our physician colleagues in the field—especially out of New York—about the shortages of PPE in hospitals. He and I came out of our February 29 task force meeting determined to get the public to understand that, given the severe shortage of PPE for our healthcare workers, we all needed to make sure we weren't hoarding masks. After all, healthcare workers' risk of encountering COVID-19 was far higher than the general public's. My handwritten notes from that task force meeting, in all caps, were a reminder of what we agreed on: that the science about past coronaviruses suggested masks (as we were accustomed to using them) should be used by medical professionals but *not* recommended for the general public.[16]

Why didn't we think about cloth masks for the public? We did, but we lacked the science, supply, and experience of a disease like COVID-19 to make such a recommendation. The physicians in the room also all knew the critical importance of correct "donning and doffing" (putting and on and removing of PPE) when dealing with a highly infectious disease. Most of America had long moved past our recent experience with Ebola during the Obama administration—a situation that had many of the same testing, communication, and public policy problems and was by most accounts as poorly handled as COVID-19 was, but where the virus itself wasn't nearly as stealthy. You can see someone has Ebola—or even most common respiratory viruses like the flu— because they are highly symptomatic. For flu and other respiratory viruses, instead of telling people to wear a mask to protect themselves from a virus that may be quietly lurking in the breath of their coworker or classmate, we were telling them, "Wash your hands, cover your cough, and if you're sick, stay home." We had also learned that with Ebola, even for healthcare workers, the virus could spread without strict adherence to detail when putting on or removing gloves, gowns, and masks (in fact, the donning and doffing process was believed to be source of most healthcare-acquired Ebola infections). Our most recent global infectious disease threat had left us with the strong impression that only trained experts could adequately utilize medical PPE.

We felt we would be able to reasonably maintain control of the virus just as we had with other viruses in the past (Ebola, MERS, H1N1, and so on) as long as symptomatic people could be identified and isolated. Also, we knew that healthcare workers in the highest-risk settings couldn't get adequate PPE due to global shortages and hoarding. Though we both stated it differently (I led by talking about the lack of supporting science, and he led by highlighting the lack of supply), Dr. Fauci and I both felt we had a scientific and a moral obligation to advise the general public against using medical PPE and to save it for healthcare personnel.

And the "medical" part of this is critical—again, *we weren't considering or talking about lower-quality cloth masks.* We weren't prepared to make such a recommendation when the science as we knew it at the time didn't support it, and it would be difficult for people to attain surgical and N95 masks, especially without negatively impacting our health care response capacity. Further, unlike many Asian countries, the US had not issued a mask recommendation to the general public in our lifetimes, even during cold and flu season, so this would be (and continues to be) a seismic shift in messaging and cultural expectations for most Americans. These factors all influenced our shared belief that needed to advise the public to leave these "medical" types of masks to healthcare workers for now.

The plan was for Dr. Fauci to take the don't-mask message to the airwaves and for me to use my social media accounts to reach the masses. But all of us who spoke publicly about this decision missed conveying some important nuances. We were pleading with Americans to look out for those who were risking their lives to keep the rest of us safe. On March 1, I posted a now-infamous tweet that detractors will never let me live down. As you probably know, a tweet is limited to 280 characters—and if you tweet often, you can forget how truncated your communication can be, even when you have the option of issuing a series of tweets. The entirety of my tweet was:

"Seriously people - STOP BUYING MASKS! They are NOT effective in preventing the general public from catching #Coronavirus, but if healthcare providers can't get them to care for sick patients, it puts them and our communities at risk!"

I further clarified in my next tweet:

"They are NOT effective in preventing general public from catching #Coronavirus, but if health care providers can't get them to care for sick patients it puts them and our communities at risk!"

This tweet was followed by a third, which said:

"The best way to protect yourself and your community is with everyday preventive actions like staying home when sick and washing hands with soap and water, to help slow the spread of respiratory illness."[17]

Again, at the time *we did not know that viral transmission was primarily airborne.* We were relying on a misperception of primary droplet transmission, and limited information out of China that the virus was mainly causing symptomatic disease. And we were thinking about and referring to medical grade masks—mainly N95s—not surgical or cloth masks.

In my tweet, I did not specifically say, "Stop buying N95 masks!" (which is what I was actually most referring to), but I wish I had. Despite our recent experiences with Ebola, I also wish I had said it probably wouldn't hurt for people to go ahead and wear facial coverings such as cloth or paper masks to offer at least some protection to themselves and others. That said, again, I honestly didn't believe the science was compelling enough at the time to make that statement. I didn't think we could say "wear a face covering" and add "but leave the 'best' ones for health workers." Still, advising people to wear some type of facial covering earlier on could have helped. After all, social distancing is imperfect—it can be difficult to maintain an adequate distance from others at all times, especially when you're a frontline worker. That said, the fact that one can't practice perfect masking or social distancing doesn't mean it's worthless to try. When a virus is spread by airborne particles (or even via tiny droplets), some distance is better than none, and cloth and surgical masks, though far from perfect, offer some individual protection to the wearer and others. We now know the *best* masks for protecting ourselves and others from COVID-19 are N95 (or comparable) masks, which are shaped and constructed differently from standard surgical masks. Fitting snugly, these types of masks can stop not only droplets but also smaller "airborne" particles like that of the COVID-19 virus.

"The mask misstep cost us dearly," said former US Deputy National Security Adviser Matt Pottinger,[18] who served in the Trump administration and frequently attended White House Coronavirus Task Force meetings because he was our expert on all things China. While we would still struggle to ramp up PPE production throughout 2020, I completely agree with Matt that if we had a do-over, we should've at least tried. I also think there's an important takeaway from my screwup with the March 1 tweet: We need Mad Men helping with public health communication.

WHERE ARE THE MAD MEN?

Nabisco works with top "Mad Men" who sit around a table deciding exactly what the campaign slogans, images, and messages should be to reach the audience most likely to consume their latest flavor of Oreos. They have an entire social media team. On my staff of less than ten, I didn't have a single person who had the training and skills of advertising experts and media campaign supervisors. And as stated, I composed most of my own social media posts. Further, far from having a single "target audience," I was trying to figure out how best to sell public health advice to perhaps the most diverse country in the history of humankind. Plus, I had to do it with traditional media and social media's time and framing limitations. Even social media experts sometimes bungle a tweet or a post and end up having to retract it or apologize. It happens every day. But maybe with a bit more expertise or another set of eyes that could review postings, I could have better communicated what I was trying to convey. Maybe then I would have been less likely to be cast as a notorious flip-flopper when new information emerged. Lesson learned: *Anyone in my position would have benefited from expert communications help, and we need to ensure public health officials have that help in the future.*

It surprised me then, as it does now, that Dr. Fauci and others (the CDC, the American Medical Association, and the World Health Organization, etc.) delivered the exact same message (and with fewer caveats than I did in my tweet), yet they received far less condemnation for their statements. As a doctor, I would never consciously do anything to put a patient at greater risk. As a human, I'm imperfect, but I am willing to own up to my mistakes and learn from them.

When the information about asymptomatic spread finally broke loose from China (and from data about spread now occurring in other parts of the world, including the US), I caught hell again as I then began encouraging people to wear cloth masks. I even put out a video that went "viral," showing people how to make them at home, a video that many said was helpful. However, others attacked me for changing my advice (when everyone in public health was changing their advice to align with the newest science).

In retrospect, I believe Dr. Fauci also made a misstep here: When the mask guidance changed and he explained why we had previously taken the position on masks that we did, he focused on the fact that we had a shortage. Many people interpreted this to be an admission of a "noble lie," and he was acknowledging that he intentionally misled the public about the efficacy and importance of masks to protect his doctor friends. That wasn't the case at all. The available information at the time suggested the public was unlikely to benefit (and could even possibly be harmed) by wearing medical masks. That's the most important part of the explanation. However, healthcare workers desperately needed them (and knew how to use them properly) to stay safe and prevent our healthcare system from collapse. The latter part is what gave urgency to recommendation, but we still wouldn't have made the recommendation (or at least would have explained it differently) if the known science hadn't supported it. Yet it shows that something as subtle as how you begin your remarks can color people's perception of you, cause them to lose trust, and limit your ability to be an effective messenger moving forward.

I believe that when being interviewed, it's best to always try to lead with the science, but this wasn't easy. The questions, especially from national outlets, were more often than not framed around politics versus health and science. (How often do you ask *your* doctor, "Do you agree with what the president said about getting my colonoscopy or pap smear?") Also, many Americans don't understand that health recommendations must evolve as new discoveries are made. Further, as humans we tend to dismiss evidence that seemingly contradicts what we believe (or want to believe), and we seek out evidence that confirms we're right (scientists call this "confirmation bias"). "Leading with the science" is therefore easy to say but much harder to do, especially in a pandemic sandwiched between an impeachment trial and a presidential election, with a large slice of social justice movement on top.

Also, messengers will be imperfect, especially if they're being interviewed live or reacting in real time and not given a chance to carefully craft words with the assistance of other experts. And there are no do-overs online. Once something is posted, it exists forever, even if you attempt to edit or explain or delete the original. I've explained the reasoning for my "stop buying masks" tweet hundreds of times and eventually deleted it. Deletion is controversial because you must balance the harm of seeming like you're hiding something from the public versus the harm of people using what you previously said (irrespective of when/ why/ how you said it) out of context to foster misinformation. Whatever you decide, people will still say, "But remember when you said not to wear masks?!"

The physicians serving as directors of the NIAID (National Institute of Allergies and Infectious Diseases, which Dr. Fauci headed) and the CDC (led by Dr. Robert "Bob" Redfield) gave the same advice I did. So, why was I singled out for saying, "Stop wearing masks"?[19] I suppose there are several possible reasons. One is that when you're the surgeon general, you're held to a different standard than any other high-profile doctor. Another reason could have been the way people perceive me, from my skin color to my age to my voice (I speak in a faster-paced, East Coast manner, but like President Biden, I have long struggled with a speech impediment—mine is a lisp. Also like Joe Biden, I've been mercilessly ridiculed me for my impediment—ironically, by some of the same people who act deeply offended when conservatives raise the topic of Biden's speech). In other words, I didn't fit the mold of "America's doctor," to a lot of America. Dr. Fauci comes across as the stereotypical gentle, plain-spoken, older White male doctor, who shares his wisdom with a gravelly voice, a New York accent, and a dry wit. Dr. Redfield is an older White man, too, and a very deliberate and cautious speaker. Could these factors have influenced how people received health messages when they came from me, versus how they were perceived when coming from Drs. Fauci and Redfield?

Maybe a major issue was—and I must admit I feel this played a significant role—a politically based perception. Many assumed that Dr. Fauci was a Democrat, which helped him among Democrats, liberals, and progressives (with whom the public health community disproportionately affiliates), while because I had worked for Pence and was appointed by President Trump, many perceived me as a Republican. I was not to be given the benefit of the doubt by most Democrats (especially Black ones, many of whom were and remain my harshest critics). Left-leaning CNN and MSNBC, and reporters from the *New York Times* and *Washington Post*, missed no opportunity to criticize me or frame my comments and actions as politically motivated, often attacking not just my statements and decisions but my character and qualifications. For years, I'd been fighting against a conservative establishment that was too often quick to discredit my accomplishments as the result of affirmative action and "wokeness." I now had to defend myself and my qualifications (which include four degrees and extensive public health and policy experience) against the purported Left-leaning champions of diversity and equity. On the other hand, *Fox and Friends* and *Newsmax* loved having me on, even if they would often cut short my health messages. Meanwhile, Dr. Fauci rose to deity status on CNN and MSNBC. Again, we were almost always saying essentially the same things—frequently, verbatim. That's how strongly the optics affected people's perceptions, even though most didn't realize it and would deny it to this day.

Yet another lesson I often share with people about the pandemic is that we *must* have the courage to acknowledge our own biases in perception and where we get our information. What we think of as news is often just agenda-driven (and politically motivated) storytelling designed around the classic triad of victim, hero, and villain. If someone is cast as the heroic rescuer of victims, someone must take on the villain role. Partisanship often determines who we view as the "bad guy."

A story about mask sterilization is a good reminder of how we see what we think we are going to see—a bias that can lead to a host of problems if we aren't aware of it and working to counteract it. To address the mask shortage, President Trump raised to the task force the question others would: Could N95 masks, thought of as designed for one-time use, be sterilized? As it turns out, they could. The trick was in the logistics of getting the used masks collected, sterilized, and redistributed—yet another challenge on our list. But what proved more difficult than sterilizing the masks was cleaning them sufficiently to make health providers *believe* they were clean. Makeup worn by health care workers would stain them. As you can imagine, the recipients of masks with smudges from a previous user's cosmetics were rejected as dirty despite being scientifically proven as safe and contaminant-free. Providers simply refused to use these masks and chose to wear their own truly contaminated and dirty mask over and over again, rather than wear a newly sterilized but smudged one. Despite strong reassurances that you're misinterpreting vital information, it's hard to get past the bias that affects how you process that information. Optics are important. And what we think we see may be very different from what is reality, especially if we're wearing glasses that tint our view.

Our historical bias told us we would "see" infectious diseases spread by watching for obvious symptoms that show up quickly. Without good, up-to-date data, the full breadth and quality of COVID's spread wasn't visible—from both a scientific and human perception perspective—until the horse was already so far out of the barn it had reached people who felt certain the disease wouldn't affect them.

• CHAPTER 5 •

PROTECTING THE MOST VULNERABLE

By the time I joined the White House COVID-19 task force in late February, I knew intuitively as well as from early US data, that the elderly, the immunocompromised, and those with comorbidities would prove to be at greatest risk of hospitalization and death from the virus. Those same groups of people bear the brunt of most respiratory viral outbreaks.

I was also determined to protect my wife, Lacey, who is immunocompromised due to her metastatic melanoma and consequent treatment. No one on the task force—including the doctors—wore a mask in early February. We believed, and were in fact following, the same advice we had been giving to the public (once again illustrating there was no "noble lie" to the public about masking). However, after we later realized the extent of asymptomatic viral spread, I regularly wore a mask while at the White House. Matt Pottinger (again, he was the US Deputy National Security Adviser who described our failure to mask early on our biggest misstep) regularly wore a mask. Dr. Birx and Dr. Fauci often wore one too. But no one wore N95s—on the whole, the task force was trying to save the medical masks for healthcare workers.

We were also like many other Americans in that we felt a false sense of security. After all, we were among other affluent professionals and within the protective confines of the White House. Combine that with the peer pressure to project an image that was in accordance with the president's machismo, and it's a miracle and a blessing we didn't have an outbreak—especially as many on the task force had jobs that still required frequent travel and interactions with the public.

Task force members weren't getting screened for the virus back in the early months of 2020. PCR testing took many hours (or at that point, days) to return a result, making it impractical for surveillance testing. Additionally, our focus was on making limited PCR testing opportunities (and equipment) available where they were most needed—in healthcare settings—as soon as possible. As I mentioned, all tests initially had to be done at the CDC's Atlanta labs. That ended on March 12[20] because we were seeing an increasing number of cases that weren't travel related, and thus realized the spread was wider than previously thought. The "send it to the CDC" model was no longer practical for a nationwide response.

We had already gone down this road with Ebola testing, first doing testing only at the CDC and then moving it to state labs as we had more and more suspect cases. However, we ended up with only two Ebola cases ever being diagnosed on US soil (we had eleven total cases total, but nine were first diagnosed in Africa). Consequently, the expansion of Ebola testing wasn't seen as a lesson learned for future responses but as the latest public health example of overreaction. Though it was by dumb luck as much as anything, we prevented spread ("contained") Ebola in

America without the need for massively increased testing to diagnose cases, significant disruption in PPE supplies, or the need to create new vaccines or therapeutics. In hindsight, it's easy to say what we should have done, but the muscle memory going into COVID-19 was of warming up extensively for the game and then sitting around waiting for an opponent that never showed up.

When it came to COVID-19, private industry eventually stepped in and stepped up by developing and manufacturing tests to meet a demand that quickly outstripped CDC and local health department capacity. (Of course, companies realized they could make a lot of money by doing so.) This brings up another critical yet under-discussed crisis response truth. The FDA was accused of approving tests too slowly in an emergency (and were thereby pressured to relax Emergency Use Authorization standards). Then they were accused of not providing oversight to ensure accuracy of those tests.[21] The HHS inspector general in a 2022 report said, "FDA made calculated decisions to prioritize testing availability. . . . This meant that poorly performing tests reached the market, although how many were ultimately used or the impact on public health remains unknown."[22] There's a saying in business: "You can get it fast, cheap, or good. Choose two." With Operation Warp Speed, we paid over $12 billion to get vaccines that were both fast and good. But early on with testing, we chose fast and cheap.

Despite the quality challenges, involving private industry helped break the testing log jam. FEMA and the military helped us distribute the tests, and we went from sending out seventy-five thousand tests one week to over 2 million the next.[23] Two lessons we must remember moving forward are that as soon as an outbreak looks as though it has the potential to be more than just local/regional: *We need to convene federal, state, and private industry partners to work together to make testing widely available as the need arises. And we need to have the testing done at a state and local level, not bottlenecked at and by the CDC.*

GETTING THE TESTS OUT THERE

The task force and the administration were desperate for better data to guide us in understanding the coronavirus.[24] Negative results were just as important as positive ones, as knowing both allowed us to better understand how contagious the virus was and gauge positivity rates—a vital measure of the burden of disease in an area.

Initially we advised contact tracing of positive cases, but the simple truth is we failed long before the pandemic to fund a public health infrastructure and workforce that would be adequate for the task at hand. Contact tracing can be a great public health tool, but it's very labor intensive and requires rapid test results. Waiting weeks (as was the case for much of the US for much of 2020) on PCR results renders contact tracing moot, as it does little good to isolate someone after they've already exposed dozens (or hundreds) of others. Unfortunately, we wouldn't have good availability of rapid tests until fall of 2020.

We also typically tell people who have been "contact traced" to watch for symptoms, but what does this mean when half the people infected are asymptomatic? There are only two ways to achieve the desired results of contact tracing when you have a largely asymptomatic virus: 1) make a whole lot of people quarantine for the duration of the risk period when they may not need to, or 2) serially test those who've been exposed so you can determine if and when they contracted the virus. This will be a controversial statement to many, but I believe in hindsight that we spent a disproportionate amount of time, talent, and energy focused on contact tracing when we lacked the resources and manpower to deploy it effectively on a large scale. We needed massive numbers of contact tracers and rapid tests, a real-time data infrastructure, and a public willing (and able) to quarantine if they were found to have been exposed to the virus. Contact tracing is practical in smaller environments, like on a military base or in a hospital setting or when someone attending a family gathering later tests positive. That's why one more lesson from the pandemic is this: *Contact tracing has limited effectiveness for tracking the spread of a largely asymptomatic disease in a large community setting, unless society is willing to expend tremendous resources to deploy it very early on when containment is still feasible.*

Fortunately, the pandemic highlighted a different surveillance tool that has proven incredibly valuable yet is underused even now: sewage surveillance. Tracking the presence of a virus within a sewer system gives you a much more accurate sense of community infection rates than going by reported data from individual testing. After all, many infected people will be asymptomatic and untested, and even a large number of positive test results, especially from rapid tests, go unreported. Sewage surveillance is a great predictor of where you'll see new surges that could overwhelm hospitals (this has also proven to be useful for tracking diseases like mpox). You won't know who is responsible for sending the virus down the drain, but you'll know you're in an area of increasing cases and therefore need to consider preemptive policy actions and ready your resources for treating symptomatic cases. *We must continue to fund and scale up surveillance tools like sewage testing that provide valuable information with little ask of the general public or public health officials.*

Once the government partnered with private companies to develop and scale up production of different types of COVID-19 tests, we asked Public Health Service Rear Admiral Erica Schwartz, my deputy surgeon general, to be in charge of the HHS Community Testing Program and distribute tests where they were needed. Admiral Schwartz (an African American female who was pushed out by the new administration in a purge of the prior team) was another unheralded hero of the pandemic, who led our development of community-based testing (CBT) sites. Initially, most COVID-19 testing was done in more affluent and well-resourced areas—places that were often the opposite of the spots where the virus was hitting hardest. The CBT program was about making testing available in inner cities, marginalized communities, and places without a nearby hospital or health department.

One of the great successes of the pandemic, however, was our recognition of the role pharmacies could play in delivering diagnostic and therapeutic services to communities, especially under-resourced ones. Nine out of ten Americans live within five miles of a community pharmacy—far more than live near a hospital or doctor's office.[25] However, pre-pandemic, most Americans would have found it odd to go to a drugstore to get tested for a disease or receive a vaccination. Now, those pharmacy functions have become formalized and normalized, and people who test positive can even pick up antiviral medication before they leave the premises.

BRING ON THE MASKS

On March 8, about ten days after first joining the White House Coronavirus Task Force, I was interviewed on CNN and shared the latest on our pandemic response. I explained that we were shifting from a strategy of containment to one of mitigation. The virus was spreading faster than we could detect and contain it, and there was a real fear that we would overwhelm our hospitals—we needed to "flatten the curve." The president would end up ordering this on March 16 for fifteen days—shutting down the entire US and turning busy streets eerily quiet. It was time to think about closing schools and asking businesses to promote telework, a topic the CDC had already raised.[26] Some White House officials would continue to make statements about containment, but they were still reacting based on inadequate data and misplaced hope.

The more testing we did, the more cases we found, though persistent testing shortages meant we still didn't see or appreciate the full degree of asymptomatic cases (as most all testing was—and to this day still is—reserved for people showing symptoms). However, spread patterns and slowly increasing numbers of positive tests among asymptomatic individuals (especially in other countries who had ramped up testing more quickly) led to an increasing acknowledgment of the significance of asymptomatic spread. The WHO, the CDC, and the White House Coronavirus Task Force began discussing changing the advice to the public on face coverings. The newly emerging data convinced us to consider recommending facial coverings that might provide at least *some* amount of protection for individuals and others they encounter (that is, they could be tools for what's called "source control"). We did not yet have research to know how much protection they would provide (many argue we still don't), but a mask as a layer of protection certainly made more sense than telling people to stay home if they had symptoms, given we now knew half of infected people wouldn't have any.

We also realized that even with shutdowns, people were still visiting grocery stores, pharmacies, and so on, and that many essential workers had no choice but to interact with the public. We couldn't rely solely on social distancing or people remaining in bubbles to prevent viral spread. Touching a mask or reusing it is more problematic with a virus that is more prone to fomite spread (like the flu) than one like the coronavirus was shaping up to be. In other words, Dr. Fauci's initial concern about people "fiddling with their masks" was becoming less of a concern when balanced against increasingly acknowledged asymptomatic spread. We still needed to save medical-grade masks for health workers and honestly believed cloth masks or barriers were a reasonable recommendation for public use—remember, it would be a full two years later before the CDC would recommend public use of N95s to combat airborne spread. However, at that point, we didn't have adequate supplies of non-medical-grade masks either.

Many Americans would step up in a show of unity and patriotism when mask recommendations were altered in early April. A groundswell of people created cloth masks to sell or give away. There weren't many "feel good" moments in 2020, but grassroots efforts to create cloth masks, and local businesses adapting to make personal protective measures like hand sanitizer and face shields, were such moments. It showed that in a crisis, the American people instinctively seek to help one another—at least for a while. How I wish we could again tap into those feelings of national pride and cooperation.

The change in guidelines understandably frustrated many who didn't understand the reasons behind the shifting advice. They were unsure whether the message was to wear masks to protect themselves, others, or both—partly, that was *my* fault. I meant well, and I stand by the reasons present at the time for my admonishment to the public not to buy masks (though not the delivery). Still, of all the actions I took during my tenure, it's the one I most wish I could do over.

I also wish we had been more mindful of our optics. When people saw the president or anyone on his staff or in the administration on TV speaking publicly, they didn't see them wearing masks. Some of this was hubris. Some of it was ignorance about viral spread (both the mechanisms and the magnitude). Some of it was based on the fact that, especially later in 2020, everyone around the president and at our events had to be tested for the virus. However, even if everyone surrounding you has tested negative for COVID-19, the people seeing you at the stadium or events center or viewing you on television don't know that. (Joe Biden would make this optical mistake in his famous "COVID is over" *60 Minutes* interview in 2022.) Public figures must ask themselves, "Do I have a responsibility to model appropriate behavior, even if I feel protected for other reasons?" Further, false confidence from testing led to numerous outbreaks among DC power players during both the Trump and Biden administrations.

Having a bubble or pod of protection—having everyone around you vaccinated and recently tested as negative for COVID-19—is reassuring, but also imperfect. It's also a privilege not everyone has. Celebrities and public figures can require everyone around them to test negative before being allowed to interact with them, but the general public cannot. And we need to remember that in an infectious disease outbreak, when an invisible virus is everywhere, we can't let testing or bubbles or pods lull us into a false sense of security—which is why we all need to think of layers of protection.

Masking is inconvenient and, for some, uncomfortable or impractical. It can also be expensive (especially when hoarding and profiteering occur). Even so, I was quite surprised—especially as an anesthesiologist who has worn a mask at work for most of my adult life—at how divisive it would become. I'd hoped more people would be willing to look out for others around them—especially the vulnerable. But if *you* don't want to wear a mask, it becomes all the more important that your family and community not neglect other layers of protection like vaccinations, or isolating if you've tested positive. Looking at me, would you guess I was at high risk for hospitalization and death from COVID-19? Probably not—and that's true for many vulnerable people you may be around every day.

Because of the confusing messages about masks (along with a healthy dose of politics and opportunism), mask shaming arose. It spiraled so far out of control that we saw videos of parents aggressively harassing other parents walking their kids to school while masking, falsely claiming that mask-wearing was causing unadulterated harm to kids.[27] There were many low points in the mask wars, but for me, among the lowest was when, in March 2022, Governor Ron DeSantis of Florida (someone I'd worked with well throughout the pandemic) scolded high schoolers wearing masks while standing behind him at a press conference. He told them to take the masks off and called their masking "ridiculous" and "COVID theater."[28] One African American student kept his mask on—he later reported having a grandfather who was immunocompromised—and was asked to leave the stage by a DeSantis staffer and told he could not return until he took off his mask.[29] In other words, this Black boy was told he couldn't stand next to a White man unless he was willing to endanger his grandfather's life for the privilege. For a governor or his staff to exploit the power differential between an adult and a child was completely unacceptable. The situation was all the more troubling to me because it was a White man in the South bullying a Black teenager over a health concern. Unfortunately, however, throughout the pandemic, many people felt entitled to bully others for masking. As late as the summer of 2022, while walking through an airport, I had a Delta airlines pilot (in uniform) stop to admonish me to take off my mask and "breathe free." In all fairness, many people felt (and at times were) bullied by pro-maskers throughout the pandemic, yet it seemed the call to arms quickly went from "no mask mandates" to "shame and punish the maskers" once most of the mandates ended. An eye for an eye leaves everyone blind, yet it seems that for many, retribution and "justice," and not the original rallying cry of "personal choice," became the end goals.

You typically don't know the risk level of people in someone else's household, and some people simply wear masks to limit their exposure to allergens or to protect their lungs because they have a respiratory condition. We all have different risk factors and our own risk tolerance. What's more, there will be times when we all are more at risk of becoming infected or spreading a virus. We should remember that when someone around us is masking, it's not hurting us, and it's providing us with some protection from any infectious respiratory disease *they* might have!

I've always said public health officials must ensure the public understands the reason for any mandate before it is enacted, and public health too often failed in this regard. Yet I would hope as human beings we can agree, *no one* should feel pressured to unmask or defend their reasoning for masking.

"NO, IT'S NOT CONTAINED"

In early March, I was telling the public that we were preparing for a mitigation phase in case we couldn't contain the virus.[30] The messaging from the White House had been confusing—officials had said the virus was contained or "relatively" contained, and here I was saying it wasn't. I hadn't forgotten that the original public spokesperson for the COVID-19 response, the CDC's Nancy Messonier, had seemingly been put in a media timeout weeks earlier for "alarming" the public without the hard data to back it up. Even so, I had to be honest about what we were facing. I was determined to be the Nation's Doctor, not "Trump's surgeon general," and I didn't want to have to defend or answer for everything said by anyone in the administration. Yet that was the situation I repeatedly was forced into.

Dr. Fauci and I were both finding that, after honing our message for upcoming media appearances, the president would say or tweet something (often at 4:00 a.m.) that reporters would question us about. This usually took the form of "Do you agree with the president?" or the more aggressive, "Will you condemn the president's remarks or actions?" Another critical and almost totally unrecognized point about our communications is that reporters at White House briefings and on national television are mostly political reporters or generalists who are more interested in the political angle of what is said than in the latest health advice on staying safe from the virus. They'd much rather have the headline, "Trump's Surgeon General Admits President Is Dangerously Wrong about COVID," or "Trump Contradicted By His Own Surgeon General," than "US Surgeon General Gives Tips on How to Stay Safe." An important lesson: *We need health reporters, not political reporters, asking health questions of health professionals—especially in a health crisis.*

Many politicians and policymakers on both sides of the aisle continued to express hope that, as a nation, we could contain the virus. But by late March, almost all the scientists were highly skeptical of our ability to do so. Viruses are proficient at mutating around any obstacles we create to stop them. While scientists try to learn about the virus and policymakers put up barriers to infection, you hope to work faster than the virus can adapt. And most viruses do eventually die out on their own—at least for a while. We saw that with the first two MERS cases in the US, which appeared in 2014 (the first in my home state of Indiana), and with H1N1 in 2009. While both these deadly diseases were feared as having the potential to create a global pandemic, containment bought us time. That allowed us to identify cases, develop a strategy, and slow the spread here while we worked with the international community to treat infected patients overseas and eradicate the diseases elsewhere.

With all that in mind, it still wasn't unreasonable to retain some hope about stamping out (or waiting out) the novel coronavirus. Many scientists still felt that as with many respiratory viruses, warmer weather and people moving outside would be environmental "obstacles" that would slow COVID-19, allowing us to gain the upper hand. But President Trump's optimistic musing about how it all might be gone by Easter, meant to be aspirational, played against the public health community's recommendations to practice the three C's, social distance, and get tested if you suspect you have COVID-19. Many began to gravitate towards this aspirational message and away from calls to take the virus seriously—especially as the prospect of warmer weather meant pandemic restrictions would present a bigger imposition on what often tend to be larger (albeit mostly outdoor) summer gatherings.

It also didn't help that, while we called for nationwide mitigation measures, the virus was still having a very localized and regional impact. Throughout most of 2020—even with hundreds of thousands dead—much of the country still didn't know someone who had been confirmed to have had an actual COVID-19 infection and certainly didn't know someone who had died from it. If they did know someone who had contracted it, that person was statistically far more likely to have had a mild case and recovered than to have been hospitalized. In other words, the more people gained experience with the virus, the less they were afraid of it. This failure to adapt our message to correspond with regional spread and individual risk teaches an important lesson we must take from the pandemic response: *Customize health messaging to people's realities, or risk losing your audience.*

Gradually, an increasing number of COVID-19 cases that were unrelated to travel to a hard-hit area, or couldn't be contact traced to a known case, were sending patients to hospitals and causing smaller and more remote communities to see outbreaks. It became clear that we were dealing with unprecedented and uncontrolled spread. My own in-laws became the first (or "index") cases of COVID-19 in the small rural community where my wife grew up. I both feared for their safety and worried about a PR backlash. I could see the potential for stories about the US surgeon general's family being the cause of a local outbreak. Fortunately, they all survived. Even so, one relative is potentially experiencing significant complications from long COVID, an outcome we weren't tracking early on.

ASSESSING WHO WAS MOST VULNERABLE

From the beginning, we observed that the elderly and those with underlying health conditions were at higher risk for hospitalization and death. The average age of a patient dying of COVID-19 was eighty, and for requiring medical attention, sixty.[31]

I was well aware of my vulnerability and my family's: As I mentioned, my wife, a three-time cancer survivor, is immuno-compromised, and I have multiple underlying health conditions. My older disabled brother is around crowds a lot: He spends most of his time at a big outdoor flea market near my parents' home. My younger brother—who has a history of substance use disorder and many common comorbid conditions that accompany it—had recently been released from prison. I was glad because the incarcerated faced a far higher risk of COVID-19 infection than the general public (along with nursing homes, prisons were the source of the most significant outbreaks over the early course of the pandemic). Still, I wasn't sure he was entering an environment that could provide the resources he needed to stay both sober and safe from COVID-19.

At the same time, like many people with health conditions, Lacey was having her regularly scheduled procedures and screenings delayed because of the concerns about COVID-19 and hospital overcrowding. On the one hand, I knew we had to make sure people understood that as part of our effort to "flatten the curve," hospitals could not keep serving all their usual patients. By shutting down businesses and schools, we were hoping to alleviate real and potential overcrowding of hospitals as well as burnout of healthcare workers. However, for years to come, we'll be dealing with the fallout of delayed and denied care for acute and chronic conditions unrelated to the virus. Another lesson learned from the pandemic is this: *We can't completely shut down and/or ignore all other health issues whenever a new public health crisis pops up.*

As for where resources should be directed—tests, health providers, masks and other PPE, and so on—we should have plans for protecting the most vulnerable while also recognizing that delayed procedures and medical tests can result in severe consequences. Plans to both "walk and chew gum" need to be baked into hospital and local pandemic preparedness plans in the future.

Worse yet, the people most likely to suffer from delayed routine medical care were also the ones most likely to be harmed by the virus. As I mentioned, people of color have worse health outcomes and access in the best of times, but it soon became apparent that COVID-19 was hitting their communities especially hard. We had statistical data on this as early as April 2020. Even today, White patients are more likely to get proper (and quicker) treatment than are people of color.[32] I have to credit Dr. Fauci for backing me up in urging the administration to pay closer attention to the increased vulnerability of Black and Brown communities to the virus. Unfortunately, I would face blowback from both the Right *and* the Left when I highlighted this issue (more on that later).

NURSING HOME CRISES

Nursing homes are both populated and tend to be staffed by people at higher risk for infectious diseases. CMS Administrator Verma helped compel nursing homes to report data so we could better protect patients, but an underappreciated pandemic challenge was keeping *the staff* from becoming infected. A typical nursing home aide is underpaid, a woman of color, and working in two or even three facilities to make ends meet. Aides' lifestyles and housing conditions are rarely conducive to isolation or quarantine. Nursing homes are often understaffed and offer limited paid sick days, so an aide might have symptoms suggestive of a COVID-19 infection, yet make a personal financial decision to go to work anyway—or be actively encouraged (even ordered) to come to work sick due to understaffing. By the time such a person took a test and learned they were positive (if they ever took a test), they would have often interacted with dozens of vulnerable people. No wonder the virus blazed its way through nursing homes in many states.

The more understaffed facilities became due to workers out with COVID-19, the harder it was for an individual who merely tested positive and didn't feel sick (or who felt ill yet tested negative) to say no to coming in or picking up an extra shift. Workers would worry about losing pay (or their jobs), yet they were also concerned about the well-being of their patients, who needed care. We ended up deploying military healthcare workers to relieve overtaxed nursing homes and long-term care facilities, but this was too little and too late.

One of the ways I've been advocating that we increase and improve our healthcare workforce capacity, including at nursing homes, is by better supporting community health workers. At Purdue University, we have a community health worker program created for this very reason. It identifies areas where we are under-resourced and trains people from the community to take on jobs of increasing responsibility and pay. Programs like this strengthen the community and the healthcare workforce pipeline, and it's ultimately helpful to have people from the community who speak the same language (figuratively and literally) and share cultural bonds with patients in local facilities with whom they work. But our lack of ability to protect nursing home patients, illustrated most severely by the experiences of the Cuomo administration in New York (ironically media's pandemic darlings for most of 2020) reflects how poorly we supported our extended healthcare workforce. The lesson? *We need a plan to help with nursing home staffing and care in the next crisis, and we need to support a locally based and culturally sensitive staffing pipeline, including community health workers.*

THE SILENT EPIDEMIC OF OBESITY

As we get older, we can be reluctant to acknowledge that we're not as resilient to illness and disease as we once were. Heck, I have trouble admitting I can no longer do all the same things my teenage boys can do. Recognizing that our health has worsened means admitting vulnerability, so many remain in denial. Sixty might not seem or feel old. And people may not recognize that they're not just "a little overweight" but morbidly obese. Despite our collective denial, we would be forced to reckon with the facts that America is the most obese nation on the planet and that obesity was a significant risk factor for hospitalization and death from COVID-19. This was true even if the patient didn't have prediabetes, diabetes, liver disease, or high blood pressure,[33] all of which are common with obesity. Seventy percent of Americans are overweight, and 42 percent are obese.[34] It's a topic I often spoke about as US surgeon general, but it's a thorny one not just due to denial but because of the stigma against overweight people.

I also wrestled with the question of whether the middle of a crisis was the best time to focus on a chronic issue that required a long-term solution. People have many reasons for not being able to shed pounds, but America's obesity epidemic wasn't going to change over a few weeks to months, especially during a time of tremendous stress. COVID-19 was causing many people to be sedentary and engage in stress-and-boredom eating and cooking (remember the flour shortages?).

Even so, there's a lesson here: *More quickly and consistently getting comprehensive data (including data on demographics and potential risk factors) would have alerted us earlier to who was most vulnerable and who was less at risk.* Without that data—to both guide us, and to prevent us from seeming like we were unfairly stigmatizing certain communities, we took a shotgun approach to public policy that burned us. (This data and demographics problem would happen again with the 2022 mpox outbreak.) We told everyone everywhere to shut down. The message conveyed was that everyone had an equal risk of contracting and being seriously harmed by the virus, and the public could see with their own eyes that this simply wasn't true.

In the future, *we must more quickly identify and protect those at the highest risk while not placing undue burdens on those at lower risk.* Mask-wearing should be no big deal for most people, especially if the government provides free, high-quality masks to low-income people. However, if we are talking about small children, or those who may be genuinely anxious or unable to wear a mask or may be harmed by doing so (for example, because they have speech issues), we must ask ourselves if it's really necessary to take a hard line in all circumstances. When we ask or compel people to take certain protective actions, we need to have (or be actively collecting) the data to support our ask. We now have rapid tests, adequate PPE, vaccines, and effective treatments for COVID-19 that we didn't have in early 2020. But for much of the public. it didn't seem that relaxation of COVID-19 restrictions appropriately correlated with the increasing availability of protective tools. My takeaway is this: *Going forward, we need (and can afford) to be more collaborative with people who may resist one or more of the layers of safety we'd like to see them adopt.* I'd rather work with someone to get them to choose from a menu of options than to alienate them because they refuse to consume the entire menu at once.

When considering personal risks, people need to recognize that it's okay to be frustrated by not knowing how safe a particular activity is. We also need to accept that medical professionals and the CDC simply can't offer custom advice suited for every possible situation. Every family gathering will have different guests with different risks, who've made different choices about protecting themselves and others from COVID-19, and the environment will be different as well. One guest might imply he tested negative ("I know for sure I don't have COVID!"), when the reality is his confidence comes not from a negative test but from being asymptomatic or having had COVID-19 two months previously. Another guest might have an undetected, underlying condition that puts her at high risk. Your dining room or kitchen may or may not have excellent ventilation. Your gathering planned for outside might encounter an unrelenting rainstorm. Your strategies for keeping everyone safe might not work for reasons outside your control.

We all should think in terms of layering protections on top of each other instead of one size or one intervention fits all (or that protection has to be all or none). If we do, it will be easier to make (and promote) the right choices for ourselves and our family, friends, and community. Respect each other's comfort level when it comes to infection risk, whether their risk tolerance is higher or lower than yours. But also show respect for others who may not be in a position to protect themselves.

• CHAPTER 6 •

COLLABORATIVE EFFORTS

GOOD RELATIONSHIPS ARE ESSENTIAL FOR solving big problems. As we scrambled to provide crucial resources where they were needed, in retrospect, we would have benefitted from a stronger and more direct link between Alex Azar, the secretary of the Department of Health and Human Services and Dr. Redfield, the CDC director.

From my perspective, Secretary Azar was hired to establish discipline and restore order after his predecessor Tom Price's departure. Azar had a reputation for doing so as president of Eli Lilly. I got along fine with him and found him approachable when I'd run into him in the halls or during lunch at HHS headquarters. In contrast, Dr. Redfield was usually in Atlanta at CDC headquarters, mostly encountering Secretary Azar and the other HHS leadership only when problems arose.

The HHS secretary and CDC director need to have a solid working alliance in a crisis, but the fact that they rarely see each other *outside* of crises doesn't lend itself to a smooth and easy relationship. The problem predated the Trump administration and still exists today. Conversely, it's also a problem when the CDC director ends up spending a lot of time in DC in a crisis. The CDC is a behemoth of an organization that requires constant attention. Like all his predecessors, Dr. Redfield was continually forced to choose between maintaining day-to-day oversight of CDC operations in Atlanta and being involved in high-level conversations and relationship-building with departmental power players in DC.

Some have suggested that the CDC move to Washington, DC, to have a closer relationship with whatever administration is in power and facilitate better communication. Dr. Peter Hotez, professor of Pediatrics and Molecular Virology at Baylor College of Medicine and author of *Preventing the Next Pandemic*, has said that moving the CDC to DC would probably put even more pressure on it to bow to politics. He says strengthening the CDC by increasing the funding, while also addressing its problems, is necessary.[35] I agree with him on both points. The CDC's reputation suffered due to its handling of COVID-19 and many feel they were too politicized. Relocating the CDC to Washington would only increase that politicization. However, CDC leadership does need to have a more regular presence at HHS in Washington, DC, and HHS leaders need to go down to Atlanta more.

Also, the CDC needs to undergo significant cultural and structural changes, and have its funding increased in critical areas (such as data collection and public communication). It should not be put in a position of having to contemplate politically framed policy tradeoffs or be pressured to temper or distort their findings so that policymakers can more easily justify their positions or actions (a charge that the CDC has continually been accused of through Trump and Biden administrations).

It is essential to know one's strengths and weaknesses and to be honest about them. The CDC doesn't have the culture or capability to respond to a widespread and rapidly evolving national emergency. It is more of a deliberative academic entity than an action-oriented agency prepared for quick decision-making and logistics. We had been in the driver's seat on test development only to have China (and most every other wealthy nation) beat us to mass testing and distribution. Further, when the WHO and others developed a test that could be used on a larger scale, the CDC refused to use it and insisted we should wait for and use their test. This was the first (but unfortunately not the last) example of the CDC's disconnect and inability to be responsive to needs in a crisis.

WE HAVE THEM, BUT DO YOU REALLY NEED THEM?

As tests rolled out in early March, a new fear and hysteria arose: reports of potential ventilator shortages. In hindsight, we had more than enough ventilators to meet demand. Any shortages were not national but *regional* because we lacked real-time data to help us understand where deficits were, or a plan to redistribute supplies as needed.

The same was somewhat true for PPE. For every COVID-19 ward lacking sufficient masks or gowns, there was a shut-down surgery center or dentist's office with unused PPE sitting on their shelves. Also, many hospitals and states were holding onto or requesting extra supplies to shore themselves up out of fear or to reassure their constituents that the state had all they needed. Governor Andrew Cuomo of New York complained bitterly about how he was going to run out of ventilators (and everything else). He received national acclaim from much of the media for his "tough straight talk" while stoking fear about inadequate federal resources in his state and elsewhere. At the height of his fear-mongering, he told the nation that New York was in jeopardy of running out of ventilators. The truth was we had just delivered a shipment of several ventilators from the national stockpile and had photos of them sitting in a New York warehouse (a story never shared with the public).

It did the task force no good to pick fights with governors, especially ones who were media darlings and who, to be fair, were leading states that had been hit hard. Despite having exceptionally high hospitalizations, New York state never ran out of ventilators and never really came close. That's good except that every resource we sent to New York to respond to Governor Cuomo's demands and burnish his image as a "get it done" governor was a resource we weren't sending somewhere else that actually *was* running perilously low. For example, having an entire navy ship full of medical staff sent to New York limited the critical work that could be done elsewhere. An important takeaway: *we need to create an essential public health infrastructure ecosystem that includes a real-time dashboard which allows for tracking of medical resources, and we need a plan for rapid and evidence-based redistribution to areas most in need.*

MERCY AND COMFORT

Governor Cuomo was desperate to show he was working to relieve overstressed doctors and nurses in New York City's hospitals. In response, the White House decided to send a military hospital ship, the USS *Comfort* (which was docked in Norfolk, Virginia), to help.

I voiced concerns when this plan was brought up in a task force meeting. I have been on both the USS *Comfort* and its sister ship on the West Coast, the USS *Mercy*. I had previously performed anesthesia cases on board the USS *Comfort* and knew that neither ship is regularly staffed or ready to immediately launch. To deploy them, military health providers are called in from across the nation—a process that typically takes weeks to months of planning. The mission of any military branch is to take care of their own, so it's challenging (and even harmful) to pull doctors and nurses from their regular duties to serve on a hospital ship temporarily.

You also have the problem of where to dock a ship that's bigger than many cruise ships. More often than not, where the ship ends up isn't going to be close to where services are most needed, so you need a plan to transport patients back and forth. The patients are, by definition, sick, and in this case, they were possibly spreading a deadly virus. Even so, the political pressure to do something was intense, so it was decided that we would deploy the ship. California Governor Gavin Newsom was asking for help, too, so the USS *Mercy* was sent to Los Angeles.

That choice cost millions of dollars, and we pulled critical staff and resources from other places to make it happen. However, by the time the ships were ready to take on patients, both the USS *Comfort* and USS *Mercy* were of very limited use. Officially, they took on non-COVID-19 patients, but we weren't sure that those patients didn't have COVID-19, just that they hadn't tested positive (or even been tested for it) and were being treated for something else. Overcrowding had begun to ease, and hospitals didn't want to send paying patients to get free care from the government as it would reduce the hospitals' compensation. In fact, most of the standalone or overflow "COVID-19" facilities taxpayers spent hundreds of millions of dollars for ended up taking on non-COVID-19 patients with no insurance or they were used as places to keep patients who no longer needed higher levels of care but still needed to isolate. I personally visited several of these units across the country, and I can tell you from first-hand knowledge that many of them didn't take on a single patient. Ultimately, the actual number of extra beds used on the medical ships was minimal. Having them come in to save the day turned out to be anticlimactic. It seemed to have been more of a costly political exercise in proving to the public that Governor Cuomo was fighting for the people of New York and that the federal government was acting quickly and effectively to respond to his demands.

One lesson we did learn from this experience was that the health providers on the ground didn't want a ship to provide care elsewhere: They wanted staffing relief within their own institutions. Given their stress, exhausted medical workers were becoming more vulnerable to mental and physical health challenges. As I said earlier, we need to better build and support our workforce in stable times and not be so short-staffed everywhere. Once we shifted from trying to bring patients onboard ships to sending military doctors and nurses to hospitals and nursing homes to relieve exhausted staff, federal support efforts became much more helpful.

While on the topic of assistance from the uniformed services, it's worth noting that for over two hundred years, the USPHS, led operationally by the US surgeon general, has served as America's health "army." It works with the CDC, the FDA, NIH, and other federal agencies and deploys staff to respond to health crises when they arise. Who better to respond during a pandemic? However, the USPHS has been on the chopping block through several administrations, both Democratic and Republican. As mentioned earlier in this book, when I first took office in 2017, I was asked to submit proposals to the White House to decrease the size of the service significantly. I resisted, and my efforts were ironically aided by the Harvey, Irma, and Maria Category 5 hurricanes that necessitated the largest deployment of USPHS officers in history until that point (soon to be surpassed by COVID-19 deployments). When Admiral Brett Giroir was confirmed as assistant secretary for health, we now had both a four-star and a three-star admiral making the case for preserving USPHS, so we were able to steady the ship, so to speak. Even so, getting the administration—and Congress—to see the value in adequately supporting the USPHS so we can better respond to future health emergencies was, and continues to be, an uphill climb.

Unfortunately, the USPHS suffers from the same problems as the broader field of public health in general. When seas are calm, nobody thinks about why they aren't getting sick from their food or why they can safely access medical care that much of the rest of the world can't. We don't recognize that investing in health *is* investing in our economy. When a public health storm arises, inevitably, everyone wants to know why you didn't warn them, prevent it, or respond to it more quickly. COVID-19 proved to be no exception. We had only six thousand officers. For comparison, almost half a million active-duty soldiers serve in the US Army, never mind the air force, navy, or marines. Many of our officers were already providing medical care in prisons or on tribal reservations, working to track the virus at CDC, or facilitating the development and approval of treatments at the FDA. When the time arose, we had no slack to deploy the people most suited to responding to or caring for COVID-19 patients. *If you value the work that the government can do to protect public health, don't make health agencies function with minimal staffing and resources.* The ripple effects on the economy, education, and lives when crises arise negate any short-term savings from cuts.

THE POLITICIZING OF COVID-19 HEATS UP

As I tried to explain the latest COVID-19 response actions and guidance to the American public, politics was always the elephant (and the donkey) in the room. I continually tried to deflect or redirect media questions that had a political spin. Doing so didn't always play out the way I hoped. On March 8, 2020, Jake Tapper asked me on his Sunday show whether it was safe for President Trump and Bernie Sanders (then far and away the Democratic frontrunner and presumptive nominee) to be among crowds on the campaign trail.[36] Senator Sanders, who was fresh off a heart attack that many felt should have forced him out of the campaign, was a guest on the same show that morning. At the time, both Trump *and* Biden supporters would've loved my help ushering Bernie off the campaign stage. Even as the question about Trump's and Sander's safety was being posed to me, I could imagine the follow-up question that would be asked of Senator Sanders: "So, the US surgeon general says it's highly risky for you to be out campaigning, far riskier than it is for President Trump or Joe Biden. Care to comment?" (Such a statement about risk would've been completely truthful for me to make about Sanders on the heels of a recent heart attack, but one that probably would have brought me vitriol and threats, which I was starting to receive from people who saw me as an enemy of their political priorities.) I imagined the next day's headlines reading "Trump's Surgeon General Says Bernie Sanders Should Quit Campaign." I wanted to talk about how we all have to weigh our own risks and that we shouldn't presume to know other people's risks simply by looking at them, so I tried to pivot the conversation.

Admittedly, my response was a little too flippant—I said that President Trump was healthier than I was. I was hoping to lead Tapper to ask a follow-up question about my own health, so I could talk about my asthma, hypertension, and prediabetes. One of the problems with COVID-19 was that we initially (and still too often) look at risk only in terms of age or appearance. Statistically speaking, my collective comorbidities put me at higher risk for COVID-19 complications than a much older, but reasonably healthy, White male (though not one who'd recently had a heart attack). I still stand by the truth (though not the prudence) of my statement, but I should have used a different example than President Trump. I avoided a Sanders-landmine but jumped right onto a Trump one. I got sucked into the political narrative.

After times like this, *CBS Mornings* host and broadcast journalist Gayle King would often be kind enough to call and offer me feedback on how I answered questions. I was very grateful to her for taking the time to advise me. She emphasized that it was my job to be as clear, concise, and effective as possible in my communication, but also that it was the media's job to frame and control the discussion, set traps, and create the "gotcha" moments. She helped me understand how to anticipate and deal with those traps while still getting my points across. Over time, I did get better at shifting to what I wanted to talk about—health—even when interviewers were especially determined to drag me into a political controversy. Gayle's advice to remember that I didn't have to answer every question they asked, and that no matter what, I still had control over what I said in response (even if it was nothing), helped me a lot. Still, whenever I did that, people would angrily tweet at me that I was "dodging the question!" A frequent media headline was "Trump's Surgeon General Refuses to Answer Question About [the latest Trump statement/action/tweet]."

Damned if you do, damned if you don't.

WE'RE ON IT!

By the beginning of April, the fifteen days to slow the spread had passed. Now we were working on a new goal: thirty days to slow it. I still feel shutting down early on was absolutely the right thing to do. We needed a timeout to regroup and retool and for certain parts of our healthcare system to be reinforced or to recover. However, no one anticipated (or could have) how long most of America would be closed down. We certainly didn't communicate the reasoning, goals, and especially the endpoints as well as we should have.

Once schools and businesses closed, people started paying attention to COVID-19 in a big way. Not only had COVID-19 impacted every life in the country, but people had more time than ever to gorge on their preferred means of media (a pandemic plus Trump was literally the best thing ever to happen for the media—viewers/ listeners/ visitors were at historic highs). Yet many were becoming increasingly skeptical about messaging from the Trump administration. I appeared on *Good Morning America* where I explained to Robin Roberts that we were now seeing COVID-19 cases in every state—a dramatic change in just a month. I updated masking advice based on the most recent data and WHO and CDC recommendations, adding the caveat that I'd asked the CDC to look into whether if, how, and to what extent masking actually prevents transmission. I emphasized social distancing was as crucial as masking and reminded people that we still needed to conserve N95 masks for healthcare workers.[37] And while I wasn't asked about it, I was starting to wonder how necessary it was for the public to continue taking measures such as disinfecting their groceries and mail before bringing them into the house. It all seems clear in hindsight, but there was so much we still didn't know then—at least not for certain—despite the need to give the public advice on what to do. The lack of accurate, comprehensive, and real-time data on which to base and explain guidance was hurting our response and our credibility.

Many challenges lay ahead, but based on feedback from Dr. Fauci and the NIH, we were increasingly hopeful for a vaccine. However, Dr. Fauci said in February 2020 that it could be eighteen to twenty-four months before one was ready, a scenario many doubted as far too optimistic.[38] Could we hold off both the virus and the public—who were only going to stay home for so long—until a vaccine was ready?

In the meantime, and based on requests from myself and other doctors on the COVID-19 task force, Vice President Pence assured people they need not worry about costs, that testing would be fully covered, and there would be no copays for COVID-19 treatment. This was partly because I had been sharing with the task force equity and access concerns I'd gathered from meeting with minority groups and marginalized communities. We knew many Americans were uninsured or under-insured and thus more afraid of getting a huge medical bill in the mail than of an invisible virus that hadn't harmed anyone *they* knew yet. Many feared losing their jobs due to missed work, or being hospitalized when our understanding of what treatments were effective had not yet coalesced into clear practice guidelines (for instance we later learned that we were actually harming many people by putting them on ventilators). "We have the tools" is a phrase that is still drastically overstated and overused today, but back then, one thing was certain: we did *not* have the tools—including the data—to protect our country—especially the most vulnerable.

Congress had passed emergency legislation to ease economic burdens on those who couldn't work remotely, something I'd argued to the task force was critical, based on my experiences growing up barely above the poverty line. I knew that would go a long way in helping people to stay home, whether to protect other or themselves. What I didn't know was that my effectiveness at communicating to the American public was about to take a significant hit—a situation that blindsided me, and that made me seriously consider whether I should continue in my role as the Nation's Doctor.

• CHAPTER 7 •

THE SKUNK IN THE ROOM

"I WAS THE SKUNK IN the room," was a phrase Dr. Fauci often invoked when discussing how he would sometimes become a particularly irritating obstacle to administration thinking or messaging. All the doctors on the task force would take turns being the "skunk." Mine would come in March and April—with a tremendous and unexpected cost.

I wanted to make the public aware of emerging data on how COVID-19 was having a differential and particularly detrimental impact on communities of color. From the earliest days of the pandemic, I had been working with the NAACP, the National Medical Association (founded to represent Black physicians and patients), and leaders such as the Reverend Jesse Jackson to raise attention to what we already foresaw would be coming. (A quick aside: once, while on the phone with Reverend Jackson, he knew I was feeling down. He told me being in a position of influence can be lonely, especially as a Black man, and that Dr. King would be proud of the work I was doing, even if others didn't recognize it. I'll never forget that. He then ordered me to conference in my mother, who I told him was a big fan. It was the highlight of her life, maybe more than watching her son get sworn in as US surgeon general![39])

Back in February 2020, I had participated in an NAACP town hall meeting to help convey that we knew COVID-19 would disproportionally affect African American communities. I talked about the need for communities of color to have greater access to testing and for the public health and medical community to pay attention to greater COVID-19 death rates among Black and Brown people. Some members of the Black community seriously believed that they couldn't contract COVID-19 because of their race. After all, COVID-19 had started in China and then hit Italy before our first encounter with the virus in the US around Seattle, Washington. None of those were places with high numbers of Black people. Some thought COVID-19 was a "White man's disease" or an "Asian disease" and that black people might be spared.

An important digression: as for calling COVID-19 "the China flu" or "the Wuhan virus," new diseases can emerge anywhere. I brought up to people within the White House the importance of the president and other communicators using neutral language despite the virus's geopolitical origin. Many immediately jumped to calling the president racist, which only further entrenched him in his beliefs and actions. However, the field of medicine has a long history of naming viruses in stigmatizing ways: by their place of origin (the Spanish flu or the Marburg virus, for example) or a name that implies an origin (like mpox, which the WHO renamed after determining that "monkeypox" was causing people to be stigmatized as associated with monkeys and Africa).[40] I remember President Trump saying in a meeting, "Well, it's from China, so what's wrong with calling it the China virus? Why is being honest, racist?" He had a point, but I explained that research shows when you name a virus or disease after a country or city, too often harm comes to people who live in that place (or whose ancestors did) or who simply look like they might have some connection to the locale.[41]

The president seemed to understand the problem. Growing up in the South, I've met people who are quite proud of their racism. I genuinely believe the president felt he was not being racist. Far from being proud, he would get truly offended when people accused him of being a bigot. However, the more people attacked him, the more defensive he became about what he felt was hypocrisy by those within the public health community—people who tend to lean Left and had largely made clear they didn't want him to win the upcoming election. He would point out their hypocrisy: the medical community has a long history of such names, so (in his mind) if he was racist, so were they. He (and his supporters) felt the outcry was far more about attacking the person saying it, than concern about what was said. He would use their hypocrisy as justification for his refusal to change course. At a June rally, President Trump would fire up the crowd by sneering at the use of "COVID-19" instead of "the Chinese virus" and would even use the term "kung flu" (which was clearly offensive, but we all know when Donald Trump feels attacked, he punches back ten times as hard). He had to have been aware of the potential consequences of that sort of rhetoric after our task force conversations about terminology,[42] and research shows that regardless of intent, President Trump's words likely contributed to the rising violence against Asian Americans which increased dramatically starting in early 2020. As disturbing as this chapter in the COVID-19 story is, at least one positive lesson came from it: *Donald Trump and COVID-19 forced the medical community to reckon with our problem of naming diseases in ways that stigmatize people.*

THE TRUTH HURTS

My first experience as the "skunk" came on March 23. Around midnight the night before, President Trump tweeted "We cannot let the cure be worse than the problem itself. At the end of the fifteen-day period, we will make a decision as to which way we want to go," which I learned about the next morning being interviewed on *The Today Show* live on the air.[43] I told viewers what I honestly believed, based on the data we had; "This week, it's gonna get bad." I expressed concern about people crowding together on beaches and in bars during spring break. We were eight days into "stop the spread," and I warned everyone that current COVID-19 infections and death numbers reflected what happened two weeks before, urging everyone to stay home if they could.[44]

That day, the Dow Jones Industrial Average (the Dow) closed 4.6 percent lower[45] despite the Federal Reserve pumping money into the stock market[46] and Senator Chuck Schumer saying that Congress was making progress on a stimulus bill.[47] Before I left my office, the White House told me not to come in person to task force meetings anymore and to call in remotely instead. Coincidence?

Initially, the number of task force members had been relatively small, but as more experts on health and policy and politics were invited to attend, the room became quite crowded. Soon, we had a spillover room connected by video and seating charts that left an empty seat between attendees. Meeting attendees always insisted they needed to be in the main room, knowing how hard it was to catch the vice president's eye or edge your way into the conversation otherwise. I had already wondered whether it was worth it to put myself (and my family) at daily risk of COVID-19 for the sake of being at the table. I was safer attending remotely, but having a much harder time making crucial points about how to keep the country safe. It had become clear to me that some in the White House were uninterested in (and annoyed at?) my advice and messaging. I tried not to take it personally. My job was to protect the people, and their job was to protect the President. Every surgeon general in every administration has had times when those two goals didn't align, and they "pissed off the White House."

Becoming the "skunk" had temporarily impacted my ability to be an effective advocate, but it was my turn next at being the "skunk" in the room that most detrimentally impacted my ability to do my job.

SEEKING ADVICE FROM LEADERS OF COLOR

The White House communications team was skittish about the prospect of speaking directly to the problem of communities of color being disproportionately impacted by COVID-19. The task force was truly concerned about this issue and were taking actions to address it, but the comms folks felt that highlighting the issue in the media was less likely to be appreciated than to invite attacks. After all, many prominent advocates from communities of color criticized the president and the administration almost nonstop for what they saw as indifference and inattention to their constituencies. Vice President Pence, however, cared more about getting the word out than any potential blowback. He was a valuable ally in my endeavors to convince the White House communications team that we needed to lead on this issue. Still, despite my assurances to the contrary, the administration's concerns would prove to be prescient.

When President Trump first decided we needed to have the task force at press briefings, I began reaching out to leaders of color to ask them what I should say if invited to address the nation about COVID-19 racial disparities. I spoke with the president of the NAACP, General Colin Powell, Reverend Jesse Jackson, and many others. They all offered advice on how to speak to the COVID-19 situation on the ground (and they all criticized the president and administration). They shared their guidance on how to meet the many challenges of being an African American leader in the public eye, especially when dealing with a crisis. We discussed the weight of representing so many constituencies and my messaging challenges, and I much appreciated those conversations.

In April, Vice President Pence decided, against some of the White House communications team's wishes, that I should speak at the April 10 press conference on the topic of COVID-19 disparities. I reached out to the president of the NAACP to get his advice for a press conference in which I would be speaking about this subject. He said, among other things, "Speak to them straight, the way you'd speak to your own family. We need to tell them to do it for their 'Big Mommas'"[48]—his words, not mine!

The advice made sense to me. After all, I called my maternal grandmother Big Momma (Big Deana to be exact, because my mother's name is also Deana). Dr. Fauci's communication style is what I would call "professorial"—you never leave a presentation he's given without believing he's the smartest person in the room—but my style was more familial. I always spoke to the camera as if I was speaking directly to my "momma". After all, she was usually watching (and would call me if she didn't understand what I was saying or thought I was being too "uppity"). I wanted my community to recognize that as US surgeon general I saw them, understood them, was one of them, and wasn't going to let a room full of White people or our president forget their vulnerability and suffering. I remembered, too, that in campaign rallies for Democratic candidates (including his own back in 2008), President Obama used similar language, urging Black voters to "call your cousin Pookie" and get him out to vote (to much laughter and applause, despite not actually having a cousin Pookie himself).[49] I truly thought the Black community would praise (or at least appreciate) me for speaking up about this important issue, and for using "our" terms.

At the April 10 COVID-19 press briefing, I was invited to the podium by the leader of the free world to address millions of Americans sitting at home. It was the first time a US surgeon general would ever receive such a platform, and especially for such an issue. Many remember I said that people, especially people of color, needed to take precautions to boost their baseline health and protect themselves from COVID-19. They remember I said to do it not just for themselves but to "do it for Big Momma." What most people don't remember, or care to remember, is the *rest of what I said.* I spoke for five-and-a-half minutes, beginning by asserting that mitigation works. I mentioned my meetings with African American and Hispanic leaders and organizations, and I shared harsh truths, many of which I'd brought up on a recent NAACP town hall phone call that they had promoted:

> In New York City, Hispanics represent the majority of deaths. In Milwaukee County, Blacks are 25 percent of the population but almost 50 percent of the cases and 75 percent of the deaths.

So, what's going on? Well, it's alarming, but it's not surprising that people of color have a greater burden of chronic health conditions. African Americans and Native Americans develop high blood pressure at much younger ages. It's less likely to be under control and does greater harm to their organs. Puerto Ricans have higher rates of asthma, and Black boys are three times as likely to die of asthma as their White counterparts.

As a matter of fact, I've been carrying around an inhaler in my pocket for forty years out of fear of having a fatal asthma attack. And I hope that showing you this inhaler shows little kids with asthma all across the country that they can grow up to be surgeon general one day. But I more immediately share it so that everyone knows it doesn't matter if you look fit, if you look young, you are still at risk for getting and spreading and dying from coronavirus.

The chronic burden of medical ills is likely to make people of color, especially, less resilient to the ravages of COVID-19. And it is possible—in fact, likely—that the burden of social ills is also contributing. Social distancing and teleworking we know are critical, and you've heard Dr. Birx and Dr. Fauci talk about how they prevent the spread of coronavirus, yet only one in five African Americans and one in six Hispanics has a job that lets them work from home.

People of color are more likely to live in densely packed areas and in multigenerational housing situations, which create higher risk for spread of a highly contagious disease like COVID-19.

We tell people to wash their hands, but a study showed 30 percent of the homes on Navajo nation don't have running water. So how are they going to do that?

In summary, people of color are both more likely to be exposed to COVID-19 and to experience increased complications from it.

But let me be crystal clear: we do not think people of color are biologically or genetically predisposed to get COVID-19. There is nothing inherently wrong with you. But they are socially predisposed to coronavirus exposure and to have a higher incidence of the very diseases that put one at risk for severe complications.[50]

I explained that the administration was actively working on "targeted outreach to communities of color and increasing financial, employment, education, housing, social, and health supports so that everybody has an equal chance to be healthy," and then I said:

I want to close by saying that while your state and local health departments and those of us in public service are working day and night to help stop the spread of COVID-19 and to protect you regardless of your color, your creed, or your geography, I need you to know you are not helpless. And it's even more important that in communities of color we adhere to the task force guidelines to slow the spread. Stay at home if possible. If you must go out, maintain six feet of distance between you and everyone else, and wear a mask if you're going to be within six feet of others. Wash your hands more often than you ever dreamed possible. Avoid alcohol, tobacco, and drugs. And call your friends and family. Check in on your mother. She wants to hear from you right now.

And speaking of mothers, we need you to do this, if not for yourself, then for your abuela. Do it for your grandaddy. Do it for your Big Momma. Do it for your pop-pop. We need you to understand, especially in communities of color, we need you to step up and help stop the spread so that we can protect those who are most vulnerable. This epidemic is a tragedy, but it will be all the more tragic if we fail to recognize and address the disproportionate impact of COVID-19, and an array of other diseases and risk factors, on communities of color.

The task force and this administration are *determined* not to let that happen. The president, the vice president, has said, 'We will not let that happen.' We can't fix these issues overnight, but I promise you we will work with your communities to quickly and meaningfully move the needle in the right direction. Nothing less than the fate of our families and friends, *my* family and friends, depends on it.

In the Q and A after those remarks, an African American political reporter/White House correspondent known for sparring with Trump at press briefings asked a leading question about why the administration didn't have a plan to prevent those high death rates. After all, she pointed out, we'd known about the special vulnerabilities of communities of color for some time.

Her response was exactly what the White House had warned would happen. President Trump told the reporter we had a plan and then touted some successes: higher employment and increased healthcare access for African Americans on his watch.

The president brought me up to answer the second part of her question, but before I could speak, she said, cell phone in hand, "You've said that African Americans and Latinos should avoid alcohol, drugs, and tobacco. You also said, 'Do it for your abuela, do it for Big Momma, and Pop-Pop'—there are some people online that are already offended by that language and the idea that you're saying behaviors might be leading to these high death rates. Could you talk about whether or not people, could you, I guess, have a response for people who might be offended by the language that you used?"

What the correspondent failed to mention was that the reason "some people online" were already offended was because minutes before she asked this question, she had selectively live tweeted just the part of my remarks about "Big Momma" and my calling on people to avoid alcohol, tobacco, and drugs. She had inferred, without critical details and context, that I was victim-blaming Black and Brown communities. In other words, she lit the fire, poured gas on it, and was taking credit for pulling the fire alarm. In the process, she ignored the systemic issues I had raised *and* effectively squashed conversation about the things at-risk people could do as individuals to personally lower their chances of getting sick or dying.

I can't overstate how this interaction impacted not just administration outreach to the African American community but also the larger public discourse about baseline health and personal actions people could take to build resilience to the virus. If the US surgeon general couldn't talk about these issues without being accused of victim blaming, few others were going to try.

The power of manipulating social and other media to create a narrative can't be dismissed or downplayed. We all have to recognize how we get tricked into accepting such narratives without digging deeper for context (and at times, we run headlong and heedlessly into this behavior). It's emotionally manipulative and causes a lot of unnecessary stress, and it hurts our health.

In response to the White House correspondent's question, I explained that I had long been meeting with the NAACP, the National Medical Association, and other organizations about targeted outreach to African Americans. I said I'd intended to use "the language that is used in my family," offered examples, and said I wasn't trying to be offensive in using our shared language when connecting with our community. Also, I pointed out that when I talked to the NAACP, they had requested my help in dispelling the myth in the African American community that people can't get coronavirus if they are Black—an important point I wanted to be sure wasn't lost.

"Do you recommend that all Americans avoid alcohol, tobacco, and drug use at this time?" she asked.

"Absolutely! It's especially important for people who are at risk and with comorbidities. But yes, *all* Americans."

Too many didn't understand that people of color aren't biologically predisposed to get COVID-19, but they are *socially* predisposed to coronavirus exposure and to have a higher incidence of the very diseases that put them at risk for severe complications. I hoped people had heard me about that, but many listeners had selective hearing. At times, we all listen for a narrative that matches our beliefs and dismiss or ignore any evidence that contradicts them. The drama created by publicizing and politicizing excerpts of my remarks out of context prevented a widespread circulation of my important—and unprecedented—health equity remarks.

Though I had flown under the radar and was generally well-respected for the first two and half years of my work as US surgeon general, this was the moment many had been waiting for. It was a chance to take down one of Trump's few Black appointees and prove that nothing Trump had done—even appointing a Black US surgeon general—was a positive thing. But what was the cost to the American people and communities of color?

The backlash was swift. Representative Alexandria Ocasio-Cortez continued the distortion of my remarks while appearing on *The View*.[51] Representative Maxine Waters wrote a scathing Facebook post about me saying, among other things, that "Jerome Adams used his five minutes of fame to do Trump's dirty work and insult African Americans and other communities of color."[52] I credit her for recognizing that I spoke for five minutes, but apparently, she didn't listen to what I'd actually said!

Every modern US surgeon general has told the public to avoid alcohol, tobacco, and drug use, and advocacy groups have increasingly encouraged public health officials to draw attention to the disproportionate impact those risks have on communities of color. For example, US tobacco-use rates are historically low,[53] but African Americans, American Indians, and members of the LGBTQ+ community are disproportionately impacted.[54] My advice on avoiding alcohol, tobacco, and drug use was influenced by this, but it was especially timely given that alcohol consumption, tobacco and marijuana use, and overdoses from opioids all increased during the pandemic. I understand people being concerned about the idea of me bringing up these habits along with underlying health conditions when speaking about communities of color and not going overboard to emphasize, "Of course, this advice goes for everyone, regardless of race or ethnicity," but when reading the actual transcript, it's clear that my remarks were not singling out or blaming people of color. Some people liked that I used colloquial language to refer to relatives, and others thought I was being condescending. I get that, though most everyone who has read the full transcript of my remarks seems to understand exactly what I meant and supports me in what I said. Yet afterward, many people of color—the very people I was speaking up for—hurled vicious insults at me. "Uncle Tom," a worse insult than the dreaded n-word (ask any Black person which they'd rather be called) started trending on Twitter.

One lesson: *it's not just the message that matters but the messenger.* While I came as a health messenger, many could only view me as a political extension of the president. Partisanship is a challenge faced by all surgeons general and high-level health appointees, such as the CDC director, FDA commissioner, and so on. For example, former CDC director Rochelle Walensky was often been accused of both downplaying and overstating the pandemic risk for the sake of Biden administration politics. Her words were viewed very differently if you voted for Joe Biden versus if you voted for Donald Trump. Ultimately, she resigned after Biden announced his reelection campaign, despite acknowledging CDC mistakes and putting into motion efforts to reform the agency. Many believe her early departure was more about politics than performance.

Another lesson is this: *we must use non-stigmatizing language, but we can't shy away from discussing groups that are at high-risk for a particular disease or health problem.* Some Black Americans were extremely uncomfortable with my pointed advice about avoiding tobacco, alcohol, and drug use, but ours is a demographic most disproportionately affected by the negative effects of these lifestyle habits. Of course, we must acknowledge systemic issues that limit the opportunities some groups have to make healthy choices and public health officials need to be sensitive too, but we have to have honest conversations about what people can do to improve their health and resistance to diseases, from COVID-19 to high blood pressure. We also have to be able to talk about obesity without people becoming overly defensive about references to health risks associated with obesity. We shouldn't "body shame," but we also shouldn't pretend that obesity doesn't put you at risk for liver disease, high blood pressure, cardiac disease, and more.

Mpox is a preventable and treatable disease that, in a 2022 outbreak, had a fairly distinct at-risk population (namely, men who have sex with men). We knew who was most vulnerable and what they needed to understand and do to protect themselves, but we in public health failed to get our messages across because of worries about offending gay and bisexual men. In other words, we chose to risk people's physical health rather than risk upsetting them. Poor messaging is just one of the many COVID-19-pandemic mistakes we repeated with mpox, and I fear we'll make them again with the next infectious disease outbreak if we don't get serious about learning critical lessons from our past errors.

THE FALLOUT FROM MY BECOMING THE SKUNK

While most of America heard—and repeated ad nauseum—exaggerated and often blatantly false news stories about how I'd callously blamed people of color, some advocates in the Black community didn't feel that way. They quietly reached out to me and told me they saw the press conference and knew (and fully agreed with!) exactly what I had said. In fact, as *Politico* reported on April 20, many advocates for communities of color were now complaining that the administration was muzzling me. Which was it, I thought? Did the Black community want me to stay or to go? Though few to none spoke out on my behalf when Blacks and liberals attacked me, some seemed to recognize there was in fact value in having a Black man in the White House—even this particular White House. If I were to leave, they might lose what little access and influence they had. (And heaven forbid if Trump actually got elected for another four years!)

I would continue to appear on regional and local talk shows and news programs, focusing on those that reached under-resourced and marginalized communities.[55] Still, the national media appearances for me dried up for me for a while. Black celebrities, influencers, and journalists resisted interviewing or working with me on important topics like whether Black Americans were safe attending church or what Black people needed to know about the safety of vaccinations. I was now entrenched as "Trump's Surgeon General," and associating with me was as toxic to their brand as associating with Trump himself. This is another lesson: *while Republican administrations are often accused of a lack of outreach to communities of color—and those accusations are too often true—it frequently becomes a self-fulfilling prophecy.* You're only going to knock on an unanswered door so many times—or worse, get a door slammed in your face—before you stop trying. Some in the White House may have acted to limit my appearances to protect both me and the administration from attacks or to silence me in retaliation for pushing to speak on this issue. There was very much an "I told you so" attitude among some on the communications team. However, it wasn't just the administration that was denying me opportunities to talk about these issues, it was also my own people.

I continued to get calls from Black celebrities who wanted *personal* advice from the US surgeon general on how to stay safe regarding COVID-19: Should they call off travel or an important family gathering? Did I have advice on where they could get tested beforehand? While I gladly helped them understand their risks, none of those calls led to even a hint of public support or even acknowledgment that they knew me.

I was demoralized. I honestly understand why when Dr. Fauci, Dr. Birx, or I were available to reporters in a press conference or in a television interview, the questions would typically be more political than medical. As Gayle King had told me, they have a job to do. In future public health crises, however, I hope that regardless the politician or what they say or tweet about, the media can focus more on the life-and-death topics and less on the opportunity for an emotionally charged political scoop. The least they can do is *let health reporters ask health question of the health experts, and let the political reporters ask political questions of the politicians.*

My unfortunate, but very real, takeaway for myself is to be cautious in attempting to address communities of color when surrounded by Whites and/or conservatives, who many people of color perceive to be uncaring or hostile toward their issues. I wish I would have anticipated that some people might not understand how and why I was trying to address my people directly—because I understood both their increased risk and heightened skepticism of advice from members of the Trump administration and the public health community. That's on me. What I'm not okay with is people deliberately ignoring my actual comments about social drivers of health and systemic racism to advance a political narrative and assert that they can be advocates for people of color, but I, who have been Black my whole life, am not Black enough to do so.

Even White people sought to deny me my Blackness, calling me a traitor to my race and a mere shill for Donald Trump.

Representative Eric Swalwell, a White congressman, tweeted harsh criticisms of me (despite clearly not having all his information straight). A White Democratic leader fomenting the teardown of a Black man based on inaccurate reporting? And he indirectly supported the trending racial slur of #UncleTom: many people retweeted his ill-informed condemnation of me with that hashtag attached. Wow. It's very troubling (at least to me) when non-Black leaders act as if they are entitled to speak against Black people on behalf of other Black people. It was especially painful to be denounced by several Black celebrities and media figures who jumped at the chance to call *me* racist rather than check in with me to find out what the context of my comments was, to see whether what was being reported was true, or to even look up the transcript or the online video of my remarks.[56] I was Trump's guy, and the confirmation bias was too strong.

Vice President Pence urged me to speak to the White House correspondent who had objected to my remarks. He said that if I more fully explained that I was trying to draw attention to disparities then surely she would want to report on that. I phoned, but she was unrepentant. She had gotten what she wanted: a viral moment from a conflict she largely manufactured. I called other Black journalists who had harshly criticized my remarks. I pointed out my remarks on health equity that they ignored, and all admitted to having only reacted to *reports* of the tweet and of my remarks rather than ever checking the original transcript or video. Not even five-and-a-half minutes could be spared in the race to weigh in and pile on, even if the price was further inaccurate reporting that led to harsh character attacks on a successful

Black man. None edited their stories or issued a retraction even after admitting to me personally they were wrong.

Hoping to calm the attacks, or at least give people more context, I also called the president of the NAACP. Eventually, the organization would take down their initial tweet attacking my comments as offensive, but the president would not come out publicly to defend me or take ownership of his own advice to me to make and frame my remarks in this way. He wouldn't even publicly acknowledge he had spoken to me.[57]

Ultimately, I am far less concerned about the harm done to my reputation than the harm done to the public. One of only two Black men at the highest levels of governmental leadership at the time (the other being Dr. Carson) became almost entirely shut out from media opportunities at a time when Black and Brown audiences sorely needed an advocate and to hear from one of their own how best to protect themselves. For many, trust in me was severely eroded—based on a tweet which led to incomplete or completely inaccurate media coverage.

Lacey and my children, the main supports in my life, were gone the weekend that all the drama happened, so I was alone with all the vitriol and recrimination that was directed my way. Even worse though, they got to hear and read about it through the media. (If you're a Black person reading this book, imagine having to explain to your children over the phone what an Uncle Tom is because people are calling you that name.) I understand that I was a convenient target for the hatred many felt for Donald Trump and his administration. Still, hatred is a blunt instrument that crushes everything and everyone in its path, even those trying to do what is right. And it often causes you to unwittingly harm people you care about—sometimes even yourself. In this case the harm was not just to me, but to communities of color. The aftermath of my "Big Momma" remarks marked the lowest moment of my tenure as a public servant. I seriously contemplated quitting. But when God closes a window, a door opens. Ironically, this emotional low of my professional career led to one of my fondest memories.

I was at rock bottom that weekend, about to write my resignation letter, when I received a call from no less an absolving personage than Oprah Winfrey. She was as warm and practical in private conversation as she is on television. Oprah reminded me that no matter how ugly people's comments got, I shouldn't be so narcissistic as to think their comments were really about *me*. She told me that people were hurting, as they have been for centuries, and as the saying goes, "hurting people often hurt other people." She shared wisdom from her career—believe it or not, Oprah's show was attacked early on for catering too much to "White" audiences though few have contributed as much to Black causes as she has. She told me if I thought I could still do some good, I needed to stay, because maybe that's where God wanted me to be. She said if your heart is in the right place and you try to do the right thing, people will eventually recognize it.

The whole world was scared, and it would be unreasonable of me to think I could be a point man on such a big topic amidst such a massive crisis and not have people slam me if they thought I was slipping up.[58] So, on the advice from Oprah (as well as some much less warm and fuzzy "straight talk" from General Colin Powell), I decided to be true to myself and let the public relations chips fall where they may. The best way for me to smooth things over with the critics was to give them the only reassurance that would last: practical health advice.

I wasn't shut out of the media entirely. I'm grateful to people like talk show host Larry Elders and Steve Harvey, both of whom supported me in clarifying my remarks and offering the latest advice about protection from COVID-19. But I'd definitely taken a hit to my reputation. The "Big Momma" debacle taught me that often the public will often misconstrue what you say— unintentionally or intentionally. So you have to have a clear purpose, faith in God, tough skin, and humility to remain effective as a high-level communicator. It was a painful lesson to learn, but I am determined to apply it in my work from now on, and I hope others in positions like mine will too.

SHOULD I STAY OR SHOULD I GO?

Throughout my years as surgeon general, and even before my heart-to-hearts with Oprah and General Colin Powell, I was continually asked, "Why don't you leave?" Many of the president's actions and policies regarding the pandemic were unhelpful, unwise, and motivated by priorities other than health which made my job as surgeon general so much more difficult. I lost some credibility as a result of becoming the "skunk," and at different points, people on both the Right and the Left called for my resignation. One of the first pieces of advice I received upon taking office was to write a resignation letter and keep it in my desk drawer. Dr. Birx and I had often talked about leaving, but we supported each other in staying because we felt we had more power inside than outside the administration. Also, we both come from military backgrounds and felt a duty to serve our country. That's easy to say during peace times but much harder during war—even war with a virus.

Remember, Trump survived two impeachments. Those battles only seemed to embolden him. He ran through chiefs of staff, attorneys general, cabinet secretaries, and other aides at a breakneck pace. By the grace of God, I had survived. Leaving during the height of the battle seemed like taking the easy way out and abandoning those who couldn't speak for themselves.

Fighting for public health and for health equity inside the Trump administration was tough. I was taking both enemy and friendly fire at all times, but I've never been one to back down from a fight. I've fought for my life since I was eight years old. I didn't want health equity–related issues going unaddressed or under-addressed because some people chose to vilify anyone affiliated with the administration.

My wife, Lacey, also gave me the inspiration to stay. I was battling to retain my seat at the table and to keep my message from becoming distorted, but she was battling cancer. How could I expect her to keep fighting if I wasn't willing to?

In June 2020, I was torn between being present with her or going on the road that summer to talk about the virus. If I did the latter, I would be free of the DC media constrictions that made it very difficult to help people hear my public health message. Lacey was now able to get PET scans again, and unfortunately, they showed that the cancer had reappeared. Even so, she and I decided together that I should continue to try my best to do my job and advocate for the marginalized, and doing so meant hitting the road.

Wherever I traveled, I felt the weight of every word I uttered and every recommendation I made. I watched audiences respond to stories that opened their eyes and ears when statistics, guidelines, and policies shut them down or sent them further into their partisan corners. I empathized with everyday people I met, knowing what they were experiencing.

People's life experiences should never be dismissed or ignored, even when we're frustrated by their choices. What I was hearing on the road was "Why can't we talk about underlying conditions and people's lifestyle choices that lead to them?" Some have said COVID-19 was a pandemic of the unmasked and unvaccinated or of the old, but it's also a pandemic of the obese and the unhealthy. While some health conditions are very difficult to prevent, others aren't. I understood the anger of people who felt those who weren't masking and getting vaccinated were selfish. I also understood the anger of those who felt that public health officials were ignoring the fact that young and healthy individuals were proving to be at far lower risk for hospitalization and death from COVID-19, but were experiencing real and myriad harms from restrictive pandemic policies. The conversations I had reminded me of an essential lesson: *when people feel that they aren't allowed to talk about disparities in health and health care, or that their personal perception of risk—whether high or low—isn't being respected, they often stop participating in important conversations and grow increasingly more frustrated—and divided.*

CHOICES

The cost of my presence and advocacy for our nation was that I often couldn't be there for Lacey as she underwent treatment.

Some have accused me of being a bad husband because of some of my choices, including this one. But my decision was no different from the choices hundreds of thousands of uniformed service members (and their families) make every day in the name of protecting our nation, and that many frontline workers made during the pandemic. Again I'm grateful that Lacey fully supported me.

And it wasn't just Lacey. My mother had had a stroke early in 2020 and couldn't fully participate in rehab. I was continually concerned about bringing an infection home to Lacey. I didn't dare visit my mother to see how she was doing and didn't know what she would be like when I saw her again—if I ever saw her again. Ultimately, I'm happy to say Lacey did not get COVID-19, but she is still battling cancer. And my own "Momma" is still alive and ornery (though she's never been the same after her stroke). Those months were incredibly tough for us as a family, as they were for too many families.

The American people need highly qualified public servants from diverse backgrounds who are willing to stay to fight for them even (and especially) when they disagree with the administration in charge. It's dangerous to our democracy to bully or discourage people from public service simply because you don't like the person in charge at 1600 Pennsylvania Avenue.

Whatever criticisms might be thrown at me, I have no regrets about my service, and I have deep gratitude to Lacey and the rest of my family (none of whom were fans of Donald Trump) for encouraging me to keep doing what I was doing. I'd made my choice to serve, and I was sticking with it.

• CHAPTER 8 •

I CAN'T BREATHE

UNLIKE PEOPLE IN MANY ASIAN countries, Americans haven't been (and still aren't) acclimated to mask-wearing during respiratory disease outbreaks. Add the fact that rapidly emerging data about a once-in-a-century virus often led to health recommendation whiplash, and it wasn't surprising that so many questioned and resisted wearing masks. What I didn't expect, and in hindsight probably should have, was the politicizing of mask-wearing (something that would be echoed later in 2020 by the politicizing of vaccines).

The mask politicizing was probably inevitable given Donald Trump's brand. Back when running for president in 2016, he positioned himself as being manly and vigorous in comparison to both "Little" Marco Rubio (remember the debate about hand size?)[59] and "weak" Hillary Clinton (whom he criticized for nearly fainting in public when she had pneumonia).[60] The "strong man leader" was an effective narrative for Donald Trump: his promise to America was always to be the tough guy who would stand up for us against China, North Korea, and any new enemies to emerge. His persona on *The Apprentice* was the ultimate tough boss, unafraid to confront and fire people, and he was further emboldened after surviving impeachment. The election-choice

Trump framed for Americans in 2020 was of himself as a leader boldly confronting an invisible virus versus Joe Biden as a frightened, feeble, old man hiding double-masked in his basement. Biden mostly campaigned from home to stay safe,[61] and despite Trump's negative branding of him, by June, Biden was making significant headway in the polls—a point not lost on political pundits of either campaign.[62] This both infuriated and further entrenched Trump. He was like a ferocious boxer who couldn't land a punch because his opponent kept running away. He believed that in a "fair" fight in view of the public, he'd crush Biden. The situation made him even more determined to highlight the cowardice he felt Joe Biden was displaying. In his mind, Biden was overstating the threat of COVID-19 as an "excuse" not to engage.

COVID-19 policies were top of mind for most of America. With highly competitive political races across the country hitting full stride, the political weaponizing of COVID-19 to gain or express support for one candidate or party over another heated up. Trump, a master at branding, branded Joe Biden just as he had done to many of his enemies in the past. When in 2020, President Trump said you could choose whether or not to wear a mask, and then mocked Joe Biden for his choice, many picked up on the strong-versus-cowardly, individualistic-versus-conformist message, especially men and libertarians.

It's no surprise that it was common to see more women than men masking. On social media, men sneered at wearing "face diapers," and libertarians and conservatives often insisted that expecting people to mask to protect their neighbors was an attack on the Constitution itself. (One study found that men were much more likely to view face masks as infringing on their independence, while women were more likely to say they were uncomfortable.)[63] At one point, I suggested to the president and his staff that he pass out masks at rallies that said TRUMP 2020 or MAGA. As a doctor, I didn't care what the masks said, so long as people were using them. I remember a twinkle in his eye for a second (Donald Trump rarely misses an opportunity to put his name on something), but my suggestion was then quickly dismissed. The Trump campaign team was not going to give up the strongman narrative or the optics in support of it.

What's especially sad about the pitting of manliness versus masking is that, just as it is for many diseases and risk factors, the death rate from COVID-19 is higher among men than women. Trump helped feed this toxic masculinity—something that had been a problem for public health long before Trump and causes more men than women to die of everything from car accidents to shootings (both murders and suicides) to acute alcohol poisoning. This disproportionately male refusal to take protective measures surely had some effect on pandemic gender disparities. More people taking precautions would have helped save lives from COVID-19, but our public health message was up against some powerful and long-standing branding that was accentuated by, but predated, the pandemic.[64] Public safety was pitted against individual freedom and machismo, and a health debate morphed into a political one (and vice versa).

Masking in public, both indoors and outdoors, would become an increasingly contentious topic as a series of warm, sunny days opened the door to the summer of 2020. However, it wasn't Donald Trump but a horrendous event around Memorial

Day weekend that would lead to the most sudden increase in large gatherings of people that year.

"I CAN'T BREATHE"

I couldn't watch it in its entirety. The violence was too visceral. The video, filmed by a seventeen-year-old witness named Darnella Frazier, depicted the brutal killing of a Black man named George Floyd. A crowd of people gathered and shouted in vain for the police to show mercy as Mr. Floyd was held down by four police officers and slowly suffocated over the course of nine agonizing minutes.

More than most, I can personally relate to what it feels like when you're a Black man who can't breathe. As a lifelong asthmatic, I've experienced that same frightful feeling on and off since childhood. The horror of not being able to draw in a breath and pleading for your mother to help, well, that literally *was* me. Further, that Black man on the ground begging the police to spare his life and gasping out, "I can't breathe!" could have been my brother, who has been arrested several times due to his substance use disorder, or any number of my other male relatives who've had confrontations with the police.

A situation I identified with even more as an adult, however, is Ahmaud Arbery's. I have jogged past many a house undergoing construction in my almost entirely White neighborhood, and peeked in out of curiosity. What is the floor plan? How big is the master bedroom? My wife and I have often talked about what unique aspects our neighbors are adding to their new homes and mused about what home projects we might want to take on. This is something many of you reading this book have done or can identify with. However, since Ahmaud Arbery was killed for doing something I, and many of my White neighbors, do regularly, I have never again tarried in front of a house undergoing construction.

Black people, no matter how educated they are or how much money they make, experience things that White people just don't (what some call "microaggressions"). I've had store security follow me for no discernable reason other than the color of my skin. I've lived in affluent neighborhoods where White housewives have boasted blithely about "tearing into a police officer" for pulling them over or about how they flat out refused to cooperate with them until the officer relented. Black men like me don't have that option, regardless of how rude or degrading the police are. You comply—quickly, quietly, and often in a humiliating fashion—or you die. And as Ahmaud Arbery and Trayvon Martin found, it doesn't even have to be an actual police officer stopping you: it can just be an empowered non-Black male playacting the role of a law enforcement officer.

Without my uniform or white coat, I am just another Black man in the eyes of police officers like the ones in the George Floyd video, seen as a dangerous suspect first instead of as a citizen with rights. I'd had enough unpleasant encounters with security and police officers who treated me disrespectfully and even menacingly to know that.

Despite the treatment Black people—especially Black men—have received in this country, I believe it's my responsibility as a physician to try and find common ground with people whenever possible, regardless of our notable differences. Doctors don't have the luxury of choosing their patients, and we take an oath to care for everyone, without bias.

Several years ago, I had to put EKG pads on a patient who was about to undergo surgery. He was around my age, and as I explained why we needed to do an EKG, he became nervous when I tried to pull down the sheet that was unusually high over his hospital gown. As I lowered it, I saw swastika tattoos on his biceps and forearms. I managed not to show any response as I finished my sentence. Seeing that one tattoo seemed to commemorate the birth of a child, I got an idea.

"So…how many kids do you have?" I asked.

He started talking about his daughter, I started talking about my own kids, and soon, I saw him relax a bit. We got through the surgery okay, and I said nothing about the swastikas. I hope that by not reacting as he'd expected, I showed him that maybe there were some errors in his thinking. Had I treated him harshly, it would've just fed into whatever ugly stereotypes he had of Black people. Any display of disdain or hate from me would've only served, in his mind, to justify his. I hope you take the point I'm trying to communicate here: that when it comes family and health, even a Black man and a neo-Nazi can find common ground. That mindset served me well throughout some difficult times in hospitals and in my time in public service. In a situation where I'm confronted with someone's hateful beliefs, I try to give them the benefit of the doubt (if I can do it safely) and assume that, as with most all humans, we have more in common than we have differences. I'd rather give people like my swastika-tattooed patient a chance (and a reason) to rethink their position than assume there's no hope of a small act of humanity having an effect that may someday lead to a bigger change.

SHOULD I SPEAK UP?

The George Floyd video left me both angry and anguished. I had a sinking feeling that nothing would change, that, once again, blatant police brutality that had snuffed out a Black man's life would lead to thoughts, prayers, and calls to let the legal process play out but would not transform policing in any way.

I knew that throngs of people would likely take to the streets in protest. I felt what they were feeling. How could everyday life go on as usual after such indisputable evidence of a blatant, cold-blooded murder of yet another Black man at the hands of police officers? These officers seemed to have no sense of humanity, and like many others, I felt they would likely face no accountability.

I tried to process what this meant for me, both personally and professionally. As a dad, I thought about my teenage boys, one of whom is taller than me now. How does the world see them? Do people pick up on what I see: Goofy boys who bear-hug their mom, cuddle with their two fluff-ball dogs, and tease their kid sister? Or do they see them as a potential threat? As the US surgeon general, I thought about the mental health impacts of such a traumatizing video. I knew that almost everyone—adults and kids alike—would watch. Did I need to say or do something about that? What was my responsibility as a father? A physician? A prominent Black man? Would speaking out fan the flames of volatility? I had already been publicly flogged and shunned by members of the Black community who had all but told me I wasn't Black enough to speak from a personal perspective on such issues because I was part of the Trump administration. Was I up for facing that again?

As a government official, I did have to strike a balance between speaking out as an individual and letting the official process play out. Would the US surgeon general speaking on this issue inflame the situation and cause more harm (an accusation Representative Maxine Waters faced when she encouraged protesters to "get more confrontational" if there was no guilty verdict)?[65] I hadn't even watched the entire video yet—for my own mental health, I couldn't bring myself to do it.

Discouraging public gatherings had been one clear and consistent piece of guidance from the COVID-19 task force up to this point. Democrats and those defending Joe Biden's decision to campaign mostly from his basement had, up until this point, adhered to such "common sense health advice" (though that would soon change). Consequently, and in many ways, I felt I had a responsibility as a task force member to make a statement—if not about the video than about the virus. If I were going to address the situation, I would have to do it quickly.

Thoughts whirled in my mind. What should I say, and how should I say it? I remembered how President Obama had been criticized for weighing in too quickly on the Trayvon Martin situation while it was still being investigated by police. The way I saw it: How could he have remained silent about recognizing that this young man was not all that different from the young man he had been? How could I remain silent about the murder of George Floyd?

I wondered what I would say to my kids. Unlike me, they were growing up in a world where news is ubiquitous. I couldn't shield them from the ugly truth of what had happened. For all I knew, they had already seen the video themselves.

Father. Brother. US surgeon general. The Nation's Doctor. Black man. My various identities all had different priorities.

I spoke on the phone that night with a political advisor from my office about the potential consequences of speaking out publicly. Would the White House retaliate? I couldn't risk further losing my platform for helping Black and Brown communities.

The next morning, I decided I would speak out publicly despite the risks. At my office, I worked with the office's political advisor, Dolly, on a draft. I spent what felt like forever reading and rereading it, not just to make sure it communicated what I felt but to try to ensure it didn't communicate something that could be used against me. Then, without bothering to ask permission (if this was going to be my *Apprentice* moment, then so be it), I posted on Facebook and Twitter.

Seeing my Facebook post, a *Politico* reporter named Dan Diamond reached out to request an interview. To my surprise, I was cleared by the White House to speak further. Given *Politico's* reputation for being critical of the administration, I don't think that would have happened had it not been for my pushing forward with my social media post—one that many in the public received with gratitude and empathy. I'm sure few, if any, of those who read my posts expected a Trump administration official to speak in such a raw and unfiltered way about this clear act of racism.

Of course, some people reacted badly to what I said, especially those on the Right who had been condemned for their gatherings at Trump rallies and now wanted the Nation's Doctor to issue a full-throated condemnation of the Black Lives Matter gatherings. Still, I was surprised and buoyed by all those—including many conservatives—who thanked me for speaking up.

In the end, I was glad I wrote and shared the statement. Protest is as American as can be. The problem (and the lesson), however, is that, while deciding if when to exercise our freedom of expression and right to protest is a very personal matter, viruses don't care about your reasons for doing it. So, from a purely medical standpoint, it wasn't (and isn't) my place to judge those personal decisions. That's why I wanted to be sure that the crowds out there exercising their right to express their outrage, whether in defense of social justice for all Americans or in a quest to "Make America Great Again," were doing so as safely as possible.

Lacey felt strongly that our kids should see the protests, so we talked to them about what was happening and why. We wanted them to understand that we have a right to protest and assemble but also a responsibility to be peaceful and act in ways that support our own and others' safety. Marching in the streets always involves some risks—sometimes it's COVID-19, sometimes it's pepper spray—which is not what someone with asthma wants to encounter, so I had to factor in that possibility. We would go to HHS headquarters right off the mall in Washington, DC, where I watched the George Floyd protests and, later, the January 6 riots happen right outside my office window. Lacey and I decided that if the situation felt as if it were becoming dangerous, we could head to safety in my building.

So, on June 6, the five of us went to see the protests in downtown DC along with Dolly, who was in her early twenties, White, and Republican. Her determination to make a statement with her presence was a real-life lesson to my kids about not judging others based on politics. Don't assume you don't have allies; they can often show up in places you don't expect. Dolly's presence offered this message, and I'll always be grateful to her for that.

Being out there and seeing all the people voicing their frustration helped diminish some of my feelings of powerlessness. I thought about how the words "I can't breathe" had been, for most of my professional life, and especially for most of 2020, associated with people in hospitals and on ventilators. Now, it was a rallying cry for people who took to the streets to be heard and express their anguish.

BERATED BY A ROCK STAR, AN AVENGER, A KING OF COMEDY, AND A MASTER CHEF

Growing up in the 1980s in a predominantly White, mostly rural community, it was hard not to know the rock band Guns N' Roses. They were part of the soundtrack of my youth, and I could sing the lyrics to most of their songs, including, "Welcome to the Jungle," "Sweet Child of Mine," and "Paradise City." (In the lyrics of that one, Axl Rose ironically both references the surgeon general and speaks of having difficulty breathing.) As an adult, I certainly didn't expect my public health journey to include a very public fight with one of the band's founding members. But my tenure as surgeon general was about to take yet another strange turn.

Science has always been about nuance, and it constantly evolves. Yet any appearance in the media of hesitation, inconsistency, or trying to have it both ways is sure to get you pounced on—especially when politics are involved. Critics on the Left were convinced the administration was not taking the crisis seriously:

it was literally their predominant campaign message. Critics on the Right resented regulations and mandates. They felt betrayed by a Republican administration that was encouraging state and local governments to mandate masks, keep schools closed, and invoke economically burdensome business closures.

By July 2020, with estimated COVID-19 deaths over two hundred thousand and NIH researchers estimating some 20 million cases of COVID-19 (most undiagnosed), much of the public was understandably in a state of alarm. With characteristic bravado, showmanship, and his trademark nod to American greatness, President Trump decided that he would speak before a big crowd at Mount Rushmore on the Fourth of July, associating himself with four past presidents hewn into its massive and famous rock. The media (the same media covering BLM protests with nary a mention of the pandemic risks of closely packed crowds in those circumstances) went berserk about the president promoting a potential "superspreader" event. Was Trump trying to get people killed? Did he not care that many of his most ardent fans, the ones most likely to show up at such an event, were resistant to masking? (One year later, President Biden declared that we'd "turned a corner on the pandemic" while hosting a large Fourth of July gathering at the White House. This was at the same time the highly contagious Delta variant of COVID-19 was ripping through the UK and in the early stages of one of our most deadly surges in the US.)

President Trump announced his plans soon after then-senator Joe Biden had officially secured the Democratic nomination for president (and while still primarily appearing on TV from his basement). Biden pledged in late June that if he won, he would issue a national mask mandate[66] (something his legal advisors would later tell him was not within his power). Still, Biden supporters were glad to contrast his electoral guarantee with Trump's words and actions.

In this volatile context, and in one of my first major network interviews since the April 10 "Big Momma" speech, I was asked about the danger of attending the president's planned events (the one at Mount Rushmore and another in Washington, DC). I was introduced as "Trump's surgeon general" by NBC's Craig Melvin, a Black reporter who started the interview by attacking me for changing my position on masking months earlier, as though Dr. Fauci and other health experts hadn't given the same advice and I hadn't thoroughly explained this scores of times already. Craig Melvin asked whether I would advise a loved one to attend.

Mindful of the trade-offs in such advice (as little in public is all-or-nothing), I said people needed to understand the risks to themselves and to others of attending such gatherings. I also said it made a big difference whether a gathering was a tightly knit indoor one or an open-air event as the Mount Rushmore gathering would be. We were now even more aware of the contrast between low transmission rates in the open air and high transmission rates in tight indoor quarters among those already sick.[67]

I was conscious of the need to not appear biased in giving health advice and knew that whatever I said to CNN and MSNBC about Trump's events, I'd soon have to defend on Fox or Newsmax when BLM protests were discussed. That's because I'd taken pains and pushed to appear on both conservative and Left-leaning news stations. (I truly can't remember ever seeing a high-level Biden administration health official on Fox or Newsmax—

one can see how "the government doesn't care about you" is such an easy sell for the media.) After all, I was the Nation's Doctor, not one political party or president's surgeon general.

In my pre-Independence Day NBC interview, I added that, "As we talk about the Fourth of July and independence, it's important to understand that if we all wear these [masks], we will actually have more independence and more freedom because more places will be able to stay open, and we'll have less spread of the disease."[68]

That's in keeping with the objective thinking of most all public health experts and even the most COVID-19-averse commentators. I did not praise mandates, frame masking as a magic force field, or speak in politically framed absolutes. I stuck with the science and explained that people must consider their individual medical risk factors and should take appropriate precautions. I said that different individuals might reach different conclusions about their tolerance for risk under the circumstances. And for displaying this objectivity, I got called a "coward" and a "POS" (that is, a "piece of shit") by Axl Rose on Twitter. "Resign," he tweeted. "U don't deserve the job or title. America deserves better."

As countless additional Rose fans and opportunists piled onto me on Twitter, I couldn't help feeling—like the title of another famous Guns N' Roses' song—that people were "Out ta Get Me." I was also derided by the likes of Don Cheadle and D.L. Hughley (who would later criticize me in his 2021 book, cherry-picking my April 10 comments and joining those who would refer to me as "Trump's surgeon general"[69]). Chef José Andrés criticized me too. As I (only half-jokingly) tell audiences, my punishment for offering the objective truth about health risk versus feeding the political narrative was that I was attacked by a rock star, an Avenger, a king of comedy, and a Michelin-star chef. These were all people I greatly admired, but the cut from Axl was the deepest. (Incidentally, I was surprised to hit it off with rocker Nikki Sixx when, as US surgeon general, I served with him on a panel on opioid misuse, so now I'm definitely more of a Mötley Crüe fan than a Guns N' Roses one!) I tweeted in reply that if Axl felt strongly about it, perhaps he should work with me to make a video urging people to wear COVID-19 masks. Axl declined my offer to use our collective bully pulpits to promote health, and I lament that I can't take credit for inspiring a new line in a Guns N' Roses song about advice from the surgeon general. However, my reply inspired him to tweet at much greater length about his feelings on the Trump administration (a "threat to democracy," he said) and the impact of my nuanced position on masking (it "caters to the irresponsibility of this administration"). This was overall more civil than "POS," so I considered my outreach and the exchange a qualified success. Plus, it illustrated that like with so many others, his real complaint wasn't with my actual health advice but with Trump and the politics of the administration.

Since the Middle Ages, healers have been driven out of town by those who deemed their work out of touch with mainstream sentiments or an inconvenience to the political and cultural desires of the masses. A "kill the messenger" mentality still has a hold on many people. I tried to keep that in mind. I was also still striving to overcome the hit to my reputation caused by my own media missteps and the partisan reaction to them earlier in the year.

Ultimately, over 4,700 Black Lives Matter protests took place, and they occurred in every state.[70] Any of these gatherings could have served as a superspreader event, although it seems that overall, the protests didn't set off a national surge (again, largely because, like Trump's Independence Day Mount Rushmore event, they occurred almost exclusively outside).[71] Many conservatives didn't understand how important it was for Black people (and their allies) to march in the streets given all the microaggressions and racism we have dealt with all our lives and all the many stories of unarmed Black men (and women) killed by police. Conversely, many liberals didn't understand (or remember, from eight years of Obama getting the rock star treatment from Democrats) how important the opportunity to be close to and hear from a president you deeply support and relate to can be to so many people.

As for me, I was actually hopeful that the heightened fear, anger, and national attention on justice in the summer of 2020 would afford me opportunities to advocate for another critical type of social justice: the form of health equity for all.

TOO MANY PEOPLE JUST TRYING TO BREATHE

What too many don't understand about health equity is that it involves both individual choices *and* social elements—including the need to acknowledge and address bias and racism. Personal responsibility matters, but far too many individuals are up against some daunting societal roadblocks to their health and longevity because of their race. Put simply, you can't make good choices if all the options placed in front of you are bad. While I can't point to exact instances of institutional and structural racism that led to me almost dying of asthma on multiple occasions, I can tell you the data shows Black people are nearly three times as likely to die of asthma compared to Whites.[72] I like to remind people of some of the more disturbing health statistics and research that can go unnoticed by people who don't live them: A recent study showed that Black children with appendicitis are prescribed less pain medication than White children are.[73] Black women are three times as likely as White women to die in childbirth.[74] Blood pressure control is 7 percent higher in non-Hispanic Whites than in Blacks,[75] and according to the American Bar Association:

> A study of 400 hospitals in the United States showed that black patients with heart disease received older, cheaper, and more conservative treatments than their white counterparts. Black patients were less likely to receive coronary bypass operations and angiography, and after surgery, they are discharged earlier from the hospital than white patients—at a stage when discharge is inappropriate. The same goes for other illnesses. Black women are less likely than white women to receive radiation therapy in conjunction with a mastectomy. In fact, they are less likely to receive mastectomies in the first place. Perhaps more disturbing is that black patients are *more likely* to receive *less desirable* treatments. The rates at which black patients have their limbs amputated is higher than those for white patients.[76]

Seeing such disparities play out in our daily lives can further impact our predisposition to hypertension, cancer, mental health problems, and more. Worse, it can discourage marginalized communities from even seeking care in the first place. I spoke with Dan Diamond on the *Politico* podcast *Pulse Check* in June 2020[77] about George Floyd's murder, the protests, and racism. I said, "If you internalize institutional and structural racism, and you don't have an outlet and you don't feel like it's going to get better, then it can manifest in ways that are harmful to your mental, emotional, and spiritual health."

Yet racism, at least in the ways most people think of it occurring, doesn't adequately describe the health inequities communities of color face. Racism risks the health and safety of Black people who interact with law enforcement, but did you know exponentially more Black and Brown individuals are killed each year by vaccine-preventable diseases like the flu than are killed by the police?[78] And why are so many minorities reticent to get vaccinations—including for the flu—even though Black people are twice as likely as White people to be hospitalized for it? (American Indians, Asians, and Hispanic non-Whites are also more likely to be hospitalized.)[79] A combination of lack of outreach and access, and a well-founded historic lack of trust, all cause or contribute to a lack of health equity. Structural and institutional policies have also been shown to disadvantage communities of color. In other words, racist health policies and institutions kill more people than racist police, and therefore *racism has long been a national health crisis.*

Coming from a very religious family, I recognized that as the pandemic raged, many people yearned to return to in-person religious services. We're social creatures who crave connection with each other, so while one person seeks a return to worship services in-person, it's important to also acknowledge another might crave a return to a music concert or a political rally. I sympathized with how frustrating and infuriating it was for people who needed that paycheck but had limits on how well they could minimize the risks to their health as they went about their work. These were people who worked hard to care for nursing home patients, drive buses, and move goods in warehouses filled with employees who may or may not have followed safety rules about masks and social distancing. Remote work wasn't an option for them, and if they had kids, who would watch them during the day with schools closed? Grandparents, who were at higher risk for COVID-19 hospitalization and death? Just as important is the other side of the coin: acknowledging that many of those same marginalized groups were the most harmed by business and school closures in communities that resisted conversations about easing restrictions, even after protective measures were far more available. In other words, George Floyd and the social justice conversations that he inspired about how our communities and society are structured were about biased policing for sure, but they were also about so much more to me, personally and professionally, and there was a lot more nuance than people acknowledge.

Until the explosion of conversations, workshops, documentaries, and books that came out after George Floyd's murder and the Black Lives Matters protests, many Americans were woefully ignorant of the systemic racism people of color are forced to navigate every day. Research on health outcomes will often reveal bias that is not only unseen but "unconscious." We'll see that group A has worse outcomes than group B despite there being no difference between the groups except for one variable, which is too often race. Diving into demographic data is extremely helpful for discovering biases that even those committed to treating others fairly can have, and *bias can be present even if you are a minority yourself*. Whatever your race or ethnicity, I encourage you to go online and take an implicit bias test; Harvard University provides several free ones that will help you recognize your biases regarding race, gender, age, and more. Awareness is the first step in eliminating biases that harm others. I hope to see CARE software, and other such algorithmic and AI-type advancements used in the medical community to give guidance on treatment, improved to counteract any unconscious biases created in the programming.[80] (Anyone developing algorithms that will determine availability of resources needs to be aware of biases that can affect people of color.)

We now know that pulse oximeters, designed for people with White skin, often overestimate blood oxygen levels in people with darker skin. That may have caused dark-skinned people to be denied care for COVID-19. They may have not been admitted despite a need for hospitalization, or the readings may have resulted in their receiving less oxygen or less intensive treatment than they actually required.[81] It also may have been the cause of delayed or denied care for me as an asthmatic youth. We lose too many persons of color due to our failure to acknowledge and address deeply rooted bias and racism in our healthcare system (and the racism is there from start to finish). Moreover, we too often fall back on the narratives of personal choice and individual responsibility without recognizing not everyone is looking at the same menu.

Sometimes, bias is deliberate, and even outright racist. Too often, Black folks have experienced the cruelty of blatant racism in health care and government policies and decisions. African Americans have not forgotten the appalling 1930s Tuskegee experiments in which the government deliberately denied Black men treatment for syphilis without their knowledge or permission to learn more about the progress of the disease. I didn't have the luxury of forgetting: these experiments, lasting over forty years, were conducted by the office of the US surgeon general. Every day I walked into my office, I passed by pictures of the men who oversaw the Tuskegee atrocities. Every. Single. Day. It's yet another reason when people asked me how I could stay, I would always answer, "How could I not?" Every day for three-and-a-half years, I was reminded of the terrible price Black people have too often paid when someone else is in charge.

Tuskegee is the most famous (or infamous) example of the government and the medical community treating African Americans' bodies as mere fodder for research. Unfortunately, it was far from the only one. In 1951, doctors at Johns Hopkins Hospital discovered that a Black woman named Henrietta Lacks had cancer. A cancer researcher in the lab found that the cells taken from her tumor could be divided multiple times without dying, which is why they became known as "immortal." Ms. Lacks died shortly after that, and neither she nor her family was notified as researchers used those cells to develop new drug treatments for everything from HIV to cancer to the polio vaccine. Biotech companies have made billions of dollars as a result (and still are to this day)! Only after many years did the family of Ms.

Lacks learn the hospital's secret about her remarkable "HeLa" cells, but they still haven't been compensated by those who profited off of her.[82] While Ms. Lacks didn't suffer from the secret research as the Tuskegee veterans did, it was another case of Black people's bodies being used as "public property" to promote the health and well-being (physical and economic) of White people.

I wish I could say such things no longer happens, but then I look at the case of the MOVE children. In 1985, the Philadelphia Police Department bombed a home in Philadelphia that served as the headquarters of MOVE, a Black liberation organization. The Philadelphia Fire Department allowed the blaze to roar through sixty-one homes, leaving eleven adults and five children dead. In 2021, it was discovered that archaeologists at Princeton University and the University of Pennsylvania had kept the remains of one of the deceased children for research purposes for decades, as if the bones were their personal property.[83]

If you didn't know it before, you now have a small taste of the deep distrust in the government and the medical community that African Americans often have. That distrust increases every time we see one of our people mistreated by the medical community. While being treated at Indiana University Health (the hospital system where I've worked for most of my career), Dr. Susan Moore, who was Black, posted a video on Facebook describing how she was treated by a White doctor when she presented with COVID-19 symptoms. Moore said her doctor dismissed her symptoms, telling her, "You're not even short of breath." "Yes, I am," Moore said in a video, which she shared on Facebook. She reported that she had to beg to receive remdesivir, an antiviral drug used to treat patients hospitalized with COVID-19.

Dr. Moore was discharged from the hospital but returned twelve hours later with a high fever and died a few weeks later. Would she have been treated that way had she been White? What's more, she was told she may have "intimidated" the staff with her knowledge of her medical condition (the old "angry Black woman" trope). It's a heartbreaking story, one all-too-familiar in the Black community.[84]

George Floyd's murder actually brought new attention to the health inequities being exposed during that same time and put some tragic wind in my sails as I traveled the country and pushed for communities of color to have greater access to testing and timely treatment. America was finally waking up to the reality that people of color were continuing to experience bias in multiple ways—including being more vulnerable to COVID-19 infection, hospitalization, and death than many other groups were—and that racism was a part of the cause.

As I stated on April 10, 2020, the number one risk for Black and Brown people experiencing hospitalization and death from COVID-19 was and continues to be social predisposition—that is, environments and circumstances that are too often beyond an individual's control. As early as March, the task force had been urging hospitals to report demographic data, including race, so that communities of color could better understand their risk, and so we could target resources more appropriately. An October 25, 2022, article in *Stat News* pointed out that "The COVID-19 pandemic reversed more than 10 years of progress made in closing the gap in life expectancy between Black and White Americans, and reduced the previous Hispanic mortality advantage by over 70 percent. Moreover, more than 200,000 American children lost their caregivers due to COVID-19—losses most concentrated among children of color."[85] The article also points out that the mental health of men and women in these racial and ethnic groups took a greater hit than that of White people,[86] and job losses were greatest among Black, Hispanic, and Asian women. While the death rate disparity has been improving,[87] there's no denying the pandemic's greater effect on these communities, nor the necessity of continued work to mitigate future impacts.

We need to do a far better job addressing the needs of communities of color and be sensitive to the fact that people in these communities have well-founded reasons to be suspicious of both medical treatments and the medical community as a whole.

BLACK MEN IN WHITE COATS

One way that's been shown to build more trust in the medical community is to increase the number of physicians from marginalized backgrounds. Fewer Black men—and Alaskan Native and Native American men and women—are attending medical school now than thirty years ago.[88] We can save lives by having more young African American men, who have a lower life expectancy than any other group, learn from and be mentored by Black doctors. As a 2021 article by Usha Lee McFarling (one of my favorite reporters on health inequities) in *Stat News* reported, "Studies show access to care and health outcomes improve when physicians more closely represent the patients they care for—partly because of increased trust. One study in Oakland showed Black male patients fared better with Black physicians because they were more likely to undergo preventive care procedures and accept flu shots."[89] Motivated by this reality and the supporting facts, I have been a part of the Black Men in White Coats initiative, which works to encourage more Black men to become doctors.[90] It's why I try to make time to speak to, mentor, or sponsor any young person of color who reaches out to me. It's a commitment that often comes at the expense of time with my own family or opportunities to generate income and wealth for us—yet another example of the aforementioned "Black tax." I do it because I know how much we need more diversity among doctors and because my family and I wouldn't be where we are today if others hadn't done the same for me.

I'd like to see more pipeline programs matching young people of color with mentors who can support them in pursuing health professions careers, whether as a doctor, nurse, pharmacist, or dentist. It's distressing to know that Black medical residents are forced out from training programs more than White residents are (a 20 percent dismissal rate compared to a 5 percent one). What's more, they often report feeling pressured by their professors to go into less lucrative specialties.[91] These are problems that medical training programs must address.

I'd also like to see a reassessment of the criteria for medical school. Historically, admissions criteria were determined primarily by White men, and research shows that it does not actually correlate with whether you will become a good doctor, especially if you are a person of color. Studies show that physicians who earn the highest MCAT scores often demonstrate an inability to empathize with and relate to their patients, and outcomes suffer. We need students who can pass the exam, of course, but who also have social intelligence and are attuned to the needs of their patients. Are they compassionate? Can they speak the predominant language of the communities in which they serve? Do they understand people who live in rural communities? An optimally functioning medical workforce should be diverse and reflect the patients being served.

• CHAPTER 9 •

THE VIRUS DOESN'T CARE ABOUT YOUR POLITICS

IN THE SUMMER OF 2020, many ultimately made the choice to gather in large groups despite concerns about the virus. The urge to travel, enjoy good weather, and socialize drove many out of isolation and quarantine. For some, the motivation was to campaign for their favorite electoral candidates. For others, it was to express anguish over George Floyd's murder. Calls for freedom from governmental restraint led too many to behave recklessly, while some communities and policy makers also clearly went overboard with onerous and poorly reasoned policies. Precautionary policies were too often left unbalanced with the need to promote mental and physical (and economic) health. Places set curfews—as if the coronavirus could tell time and only came out at night. Increasingly, we were realizing that the risk of COVID-19 infection outdoors was far smaller than indoors, yet cities chained up swing sets or wove yellow hazard tape around playground equipment to keep kids away. Huge piles of sand were dumped on one skateboard park to prevent its use.[92]

A chronic state of fear and confusion amplified the public's outrage. People across the country bristled at restrictions that made no sense to them, especially ones banning activities where people were outdoors and could socially distance. Growing anger and frustration led to heightened (and often unfair) scrutiny of public health officials, including Dr. Fauci. In late July, he was spotted in the stands at the Washington Nationals' ballpark, sitting by two other people he knew and surrounded by empty seats. Some deemed his action hypocritical—especially as so many sports parks and arenas across the country were still closed to the public. In August 2020, while in Hawaii to visit testing sites and support the Hawaii governor's and Honolulu mayor's COVID-19 response, I was ticketed for walking alone in a park on the way back from the beach. Though it was legal to be in the water, the park was closed due to COVID-19 except for those walking directly through it to access the beach. My purported crime was that I paused for thirty seconds to snap a picture of the scenery *while alone!* Though I was there on government business, the administration informed me I'd have to find and pay for my own local lawyer to defend myself against a $5,000 fine and possible jail time (after several months and the revelation of a scandal involving the officers who gave me the ticket,[93] my lawyer was eventually able to get the charges dismissed).[94] Worse, while over sixty thousand citations on the island were thrown out without legal intervention due to overzealous enforcement,[95] my citation was not.

Many news outlets gleefully reported the story as proof that "Trump's surgeon general" had carelessly endangered people. BET.com, an outlet that is proudly and loudly "pro-Black" and frequent laments the over-criminalization of Black males, pushed a headline declaring that the most prominent Black male in the administration was "facing jail time."[96] Some felt I was targeted not just by officers seeking to justify their overtime but by a legal system in a state that leans Left and where hatred of Trump is widespread.

My case dragged on over several months, requiring multiple appearances by my lawyer. I worried about the threat of incarceration hanging over my head simply for doing my job and trying to maintain my personal health in the process. This may not seem like a big deal to most readers, but for a Black man, the threat of jail feels very real and is very emotionally disturbing—especially when many of the Black males in your own family have been locked up. However, critics on both sides—those who hated Trump, and those who hated COVID-19 mitigation policies—were only too quick to tell me that I was getting exactly what I deserved. It was around this time that I needed to start taking additional medication to control my blood pressure.

I'd like all of us to take a deep breath and reflect on moments such as these and our treatment and distrust of one another. We all are responsible for reducing risks where we reasonably can but must also acknowledge we can't eliminate them entirely. As difficult as it was for everyone to keep up with the science and changing guidelines during a rapidly evolving public health crisis, neither Dr. Fauci nor I were callously putting vulnerable lives at risk during our high-profile moments outdoors that summer. Many media outlets, especially those that tended to lean Left, lightheartedly covered Dr. Fauci's incredibly errant "first pitch" (sorry, Tony, I love you, but stick to virology) without questioning his choice to attend a baseball game, while others were being severely chastised for gathering for different (often politically motivated) reasons. Those same outlets focused solely on my "incompetence" or callous endangerment of others—for literally taking a walk alone in a park. Meanwhile, outlets that leaned right attacked Fauci without acknowledging that he was outside, and social distanced (and that he was actually trying to calm public fears about the virus and show that we were beginning to reopen society—something those same outlets has been loudly calling for). It shows the challenge of being a highly visible public official and constantly needing to be hyperaware of the image one projects. People can be very unforgiving if they think you aren't practicing what you're preaching, especially when they feel they are being unduly burdened. I honestly do understand how without context, the headline, "Surgeon general cited for violating local COVID-19 ordinance" could upset people, and I very much get the terrible optics of the face of pandemic shutdowns enjoying himself at a ballgame while schools were still shut down. Yet it also shows that we need to recognize our own biases and to understand public officials are ordinary people just trying to live their lives like everyone else.

OLD SCHOOL, LITERALLY

The doctors on the task force created a side group that met outside normal task force meetings to discuss the latest research findings and the pros and cons of particular policy choices. Our group included me, Dr. Birx, Dr. Fauci, CDC director Dr. Bob Redfield, assistant secretary for health Dr. Brett Giroir, and FDA commissioner Dr. Stephen "Steve" Hahn. (By the way, people criticize the FDA's response but forget that Dr. Hahn had just begun his job in December 2019, only to get slammed immediately with both unprecedented and urgent decisions regarding testing, treatments, and vaccine production and authorization.) As fall approached, our conversations began to focus on reopening America's 130,000 or so schools,[97] many of which had closed in March and gone fully remote through the end of the school year.

Despite the binary rhetoric, we had to consider many variables and tradeoffs. We had to be sensitive to the fact that schools mere miles apart might face very different challenges. Many have argued that most teachers and students tend to be under age fifty-five[98] and thus are at lower risk for acute harm from COVID-19, so we should not have closed schools. However, many schoolchildren regularly interact with older people and others at high risk for hospitalization and death due to underlying conditions—caretakers, school bus drivers, school cafeteria workers, and so on. In fact, it's estimated over 8 million children worldwide lost a primary caregiver due to the pandemic.[99] Far too many public schools are overcrowded, meaning few had the space to have students socially distance. Moreover, too many of our nation's school buildings, especially those in poorer communities or that serve higher percentages of minorities, are old and in desperate need of repairs and upgrades. About 40 percent of our schools have problems with their HVAC systems.[100]

I still don't believe we appreciate the harms of poor ventilation, harms that predate and extend far beyond the pandemic. We have underinvested in ventilation systems in public buildings (remember, communities often use school buildings for many purposes), and on the whole, poorer people don't have the same level of access to well-ventilated working and living spaces as middle class and wealthier people do. That's reflected in the state of school buildings in low-income versus high-income areas.

Ventilation challenges, teachers not having the infrastructure or training to teach remotely, lack of high-quality (or at the time, any) masks for staff and kids, moms driving their kids to a parking lot to get broadband so they could attend school on their smart phones. It doesn't matter if you were for shutdowns or reopenings, either way, we weren't sufficiently supporting schools and students as they sought to navigate the challenges of the pandemic. Once again, the pandemic exposed longstanding obstacles to health—ones that have long disproportionately harmed Black and Brown students. (Former US surgeon general Dr. Jocelyn Elders has often said, "it's hard be healthy if you're not educated, and it's hard to be educated if you're not healthy." Our experience with schools and the pandemic showed this to be true.)

The pressure to solve the school problem was intense. Keeping schools closed would cause mounting and disproportionate educational and emotional harm even as it would protect the physical health of many vulnerable children and caregivers. The public needed clear and reasonable guidance, and the CDC was once again on the wrong side of General Colin Powell's 40/70 rule: they waited so long to issue guidance that they became irrelevant. Unfortunately, we were soon distracted by someone who had caught the president's eye and had a very fixed (and perhaps privileged) perspective on this complex issue.

TOO MUCH NOISE

Dr. Scott Atlas, a radiologist, is a senior fellow at the Hoover Institution (a conservative public policy think tank) and has advised several Republican presidential candidates during their campaigns. In the spring of 2020, he began showing up on Fox News and other conservative media outlets, where he touted the value of "natural immunity." (To be clear, "natural" immunity technically includes immunity obtained via vaccination since our immune systems naturally respond to vaccines. The antigen stimulating our immune response is manufactured, but the body responds as naturally as it does to all antigens. However, Dr. Atlas and many others imprecisely defined natural immunity as immunity acquired through infection versus vaccination.) President Trump was intrigued by Dr. Atlas's pronouncements and appointed him as an advisor to the White House Coronavirus Task Force.

Unlike others attending the meetings, Dr. Atlas had no particular or relevant experience in public health, public policy implementation, or agency expertise to share. He was a physician (though unlike others on the task force, not one who directly cared for critically ill patients) and seemed to be there primarily because he was saying things the president wanted to hear on the president's favorite news channel. Please don't misunderstand me. Raising questions and presenting contrary viewpoints is a good thing. Barack Obama famously spoke of how no one in his cabinet wanted to bring him opposing viewpoints. This made it challenging for him to obtain honest feedback on important policy decisions. We on the task force often had disagreements about how new data or a new research finding should impact our policy recommendations. As a parent myself, I wondered if many places weren't being too conservative regarding school re-openings, so I was willing to hear Dr. Atlas out. He forced conversations about school openings, and I honestly believe that had he and others not placed pressure on the CDC to more quickly adjust school guidance, schools would've remained closed a lot longer, causing further educational and emotional harm. Unfortunately, Dr. Atlas's priority (or at least his task force discussions) never seemed to be about figuring out the *safest* way to have in-person schooling—especially for the many children with chronic diseases and comorbidities. His argument always seemed to me to be more about using kids as vectors to ensure viral spread in an attempt to reach herd immunity as quickly as possible so as to reopen the economy. Worse, the danger of this approach for any vulnerable teachers, staff, or caregivers, was just considered to be acceptable collateral damage. In hindsight, put another way, people act as if the concern was always and solely about the welfare of the kids. In real time, however, most of the conversation led by Dr. Atlas and others who focused on this concept of forcing schools to open to facilitate herd immunity was about how deliberately infecting the kids would ultimately help the adults who wanted the economy open.

All the doctors on the task force considered Dr. Scott's idea for achieving herd immunity by essentially using our children as guinea pigs to be a non-starter. There was still so much we didn't know at the time (and still don't know) about short- and long-term effects of the virus. To me, the very idea was ironic, as many people criticize the idea of childhood vaccinations saying "We shouldn't experiment on our kids or ask them to carry the burden for adults." Yet those same people had no problem with the acute and chronic risks of exposing our kids to an unknown virus! We didn't yet have the tools to protect the vulnerable. And while some point to Sweden as a success story of letting COVID-19 "burn through" the population, the Swedes actually suffered more deaths and worse economic impact from their handling of the crisis than did other Scandinavian countries.[101] We also must remember that most European countries, especially those in the Scandinavian region, provide both universal access to healthcare and far more social supports (largely via higher taxes) for *all* their citizens. This underacknowledged but critically important fact helped mitigate the downsides of earlier opening in those countries.

It seemed clear from the beginning that Dr. Atlas wasn't there to have a hearty discussion or scientific debate about pros and cons, but to downplay the harms of the virus and advance an agenda. It was wearying to deal with him trying (and being allowed) to dominate the conversation with his theories at the expense of science- and experience-driven dialogue on how to best balance protecting the most vulnerable with reopening society. That balance was an extremely important consideration, especially for at-risk communities and populations, given that we had no vaccine and were desperate for effective treatments at that point. It's easy to forget that we were still at a stage where most people had no immunity, we still didn't know for sure how the virus was transmitted or all the risk factors for who would become severely ill (remember the debate over blood type?). Getting the virus still came with the very real fear of ending up on a ventilator, or worse.

Dr. Atlas was not only typically afforded more speaking time than the other doctors at task force meetings (it seemed there was an effort to ensure that his "side"—a side of one—got equal or greater time than the other side, which constituted all the other doctors in the room), but also had greater daily access to the president and White House staff. His presence went beyond a healthy discussion of competing ideas and quickly became a poisoning of the well of the scientific information the rest of the doctors were providing to the president. Dr. Birx has talked about charts and graphs the president showed her that were unfamiliar to her and were, presumably, created or found by Dr. Atlas. These were presented without context or an opposing view from others on the task force, despite ironic narratives that Dr. Atlas was the one being "shut out" of the conversation.[102]

The doctors group began spending more time discussing internal strategy—deciding, for example, that I should approach the vice president or his chief of staff about an issue we felt was being misrepresented. After all, everyone knew about my previous work and relationships with the office, and I had a closer connection to the vice president and his staff than any other doctor on the task force—besides Dr. Atlas—had to President Trump or Vice President Pence. Anyone who has worked with President Trump knows that whoever speaks to him last has the most influence and that he often makes policy decisions quickly after hearing something he agrees with. Dr. Atlas's seeming daily access to the Oval Office also coincided with a time when far fewer formal task force meetings were occurring, and we found that the other doctors' concerns were being minimized.

While I hold no ill will towards Dr. Atlas (the truth is, he and I barely conversed), his effect on President Trump and the task force demonstrates another point I often make to people who ask why I didn't "just quit." It wasn't just that I was often the only

Black/rurally raised/asthmatic person/former public health official/practicing critical care doctor/etc. in the room and that those perspectives would be lost if I left. It's that when someone leaves, it creates a vacuum, and others can fill that vacuum to gain even more influence. Once again, the question I'd ask myself (and I now ask you, the reader) is not "how could I stay?" but "how could I leave?" Representative Marcy Kaptur of Ohio, the longest-serving Democrat in the House of Representatives, has said, "So why do I stay? It isn't just to get a title. But to use every ounce of strength I have to try to hammer this message: You're leaving us out. You're not seeing us."[103] That's how I felt.

Clearly, operating solely through the White House task force was becoming less and less effective. We doctors realized we would have to find another way to influence policy at the ground level, and eventually, Dr. Birx became so fed up with Dr. Atlas that she refused to continue attending task force meetings with him. As her workspace was in the White House, she faced daily frustrations at having her opinions disregarded—I'm surprised her patience held out as long as it did.

I had already been traveling to help open testing sites across the country, but at that point, Dr. Birx suggested a fifty-state plan for meeting with governors and state health officials in person to help advance our health agenda. We would support them as they sought to apply our task force recommendations in ways that worked for their communities. We also knew that state and regional media would be far more interested in the local health story—"Surgeon General/Ambassador Birx Comes to State and Meets with Governor"—than pursuing a more nationally framed political story on Trump. In the interest of adapting our strategy to help more people in more places, Dr. Birx and I divvied up the list and hit the road.

A FIFTY-STATE TOUR

I can't emphasize enough that, given the diversity of the US (not to mention the text of the US Constitution), the federal government's job wasn't to compel the nation to adopt one-size-fits-all pandemic policies—no matter what people wanted to believe or campaigned on. Biden's unfulfilled promise of a national mask mandate was an example: it simply wasn't enforceable, legally or pragmatically. The task force's job was to provide data and guidance and to assist states in setting policies that worked best for them. What's right for a highly populous state might not work well in a smaller one, and vice versa. PPE and testing were available in some spots and not others because of disparities in population density. Los Angeles County alone has so many people that if it were a state, it would rank eleventh in population.[104] (This is yet another lesson learned: *we did not treat similarly sized populations appropriately.* The 10 million people of Los Angeles County often received fewer resources—and certainly less direct federal attention—than the 650,000 people of Vermont). Dr. Birx and I understood the need for states to customize their responses and for us to help them do it.

CDC director Redfield and FDA commissioner Hahn made a few visits to states, but they had agencies to run. Because of his work at NIAID and his age, Dr. Fauci didn't participate in the state visits, so Dr. Birx and I did most of them. In a short amount of time, I visited sites in Pennsylvania, Georgia, Florida, Maryland, Hawaii, Alabama, California, Nevada, South Carolina,

Texas, Montana, and South Dakota. So, while Dr. Fauci rightly deserves accolades for his tremendous work in the DC area and at NIH assisting with the vaccine, while he was conducting national TV interviews from his home, or office, other doctors on the task force risked their lives traveling the country prior to a vaccine or good treatments, eager to appeal directly to governors and states to adopt COVID-19 precautions and reject Dr. Atlas's calls to pursue herd immunity. This is not to diminish anything Dr. Fauci did—his contributions were remarkable—but he was part of a team of task force members who often don't get the appreciation they deserve for serving their country.

Wherever I traveled in the US, I encouraged people to get tested. I often swabbed myself on live local television, as many expressed fearing how painful a nasopharyngeal COVID-19 test swab could be. The science would evolve, showing us that a swab taken from lower in the nose was equally effective, so I then shifted to demonstrating how easy and pain-free testing had become. Still, professionals at many medical facilities (ironically, but especially US military medical staff) resisted changing their technique. This was just one of many examples of how hard it was to translate rapidly changing knowledge about the virus into broad practice, even when politics wasn't getting in the way.

We had finally gotten tests delivered to most major medical centers and urban areas, which gave the impression from a thirty-thousand-foot view that testing was widely available. Even though members of the Trump administration often repeated these assurances, our local visits revealed tests were not always going to the hardest-hit communities. I let the task force know we were having outbreaks not just in New York or New Orleans, but in remote areas, where I learned that PCR testing was all but useless for viral containment. It often took several days just to send a PCR sample from upstate tribal communities in Montana (that is, if the weather allowed the planes to fly) to the health department in Helena. Then, it took a day or more to process the test and receive the result. (I learned this after taking off from Helena on a National Guard flight and making an emergency landing in Billings because we couldn't break through the weather to land at a reservation in upstate Montana.) Making rapid tests available was imperative, and the administration was working with American companies to make that happen as quickly as possible, but it wasn't happening quickly enough. By hearing from traditionally under-resourced and overlooked communities—something that wouldn't have happened had I stayed in DC (or even stuck to the major US cities) and not made a point of visiting more disconnected areas—I was able to share their stories and expand the pool of who had access to testing.

Armed with Dr. Birx's data, I showed governors and health commissioners what their states looked like compared to the national average and helped them develop mitigation strategies that would work best for their people. Sometimes, I helped persuade governors to embrace policies that their own state health departments had been calling for but had been unable to convince their administrations to adopt. Other times, I provided cover for governors when they spoke with their local media and constituents by going over their state data and explaining the reasoning behind setting or easing strict mitigation measures. All the governors I worked with, no matter their political affiliation, expressed appreciation to us for being on the ground with them.

I praised their efforts publicly whenever I could and stood beside them and the state health commissioners to deliver a unified message showing the federal government was there to help them, not dominate them. It was grueling but often far more effective than sparring for three to five minutes on CNN or Fox morning news from a studio truck in DC.

Often, big cities and less-populated areas of the states clashed on COVID-19 policy. Sometimes governors and mayors were at odds, even when they were of the same political party. (New York governor Andrew Cuomo and New York City mayor Bill DeBlasio were prime examples.) In California, I met directly with Los Angeles mayor Eric Garcetti, who represents more people than most governors do. At one point, Dr. Birx, Dr. Fauci, and I began having weekly phone calls with southern Florida mayors. Many were Democrats serving large minority constituencies and felt they weren't getting adequate cooperation or information from the state.

Some states rightly drew a larger share of attention and funding because of their caseload, but politics and media attention also affected how much support they received (again, see New York governor Cuomo). Worse, if a Democratic governor was actively badmouthing the administration, or heaven forbid, running for office themselves, they were less likely to welcome a visit from or media appearance with a Trump political appointee (I visited and appeared with the Mayors of both New York City and LA, but neither of those state's Governors met with me).

During my visits, I tried to be bipartisan and diplomatic, often leaning on relationships I had created prior to the pandemic. (As the surgeon general, I had made it a point to alert and visit with the governor's offices and state health departments whenever I was traveling to a state. I knew the Obama administration had been criticized for not doing this during the Ebola scare of 2014.) One of my favorite governors was Democrat John Bel Edwards of Louisiana, who I thought did a great job in his state and welcomed me with open arms. Another of my favorites was Republican Larry Hogan of Maryland, who did more than most people know to help steady the ship in 2020 when he served as head of the National Governors Association. Given the primacy of states in determining health policy, the country would've had *many* more problems that year if a more politically extreme governor of either party had been at the helm. Yet despite my best intentions and attempts to be even-handed, I traveled to more red states than blue ones during the pandemic, because that's who wanted me there. Red states have always tended to suffer from poorer health status, and many of those same states also have larger percentages and absolute numbers of minorities than most coastal and Left-leaning states. Consequently, I felt that God was placing me where I was most needed. A lesson from the pandemic that we'd do well to remember is what Brian Castrucci, president and CEO of the de Beaumont Foundation, said: "Your governor has more impact on your health than your doctor does."[105] No matter what a president (or presidential candidate) tells you they will do to protect your health, more often than not, it's the governors who make the calls (think about abortion access or gun laws, or Medicaid expansion).

Despite all our visits and interactions with state health officials and governors, I regret that too often—especially early on—we didn't communicate necessary nuances about the reasoning behind federal guidance as well as we should have. And as I mentioned in an earlier chapter, we didn't always customize our guidance as well as we might have—Boise, Idaho isn't Boston, Massachusetts. But with the lack of rapid testing, we had trouble determining where viral spread was occurring and which policies were most helpful at stopping it, so we were too often overreacting in some places even as we were underreacting in others.

Much as we would all like to put COVID-19 behind us, we still need further studies on which scientific and policy interventions were most effective. That way, conversations about future guidelines can happen before we experience the next big infectious disease threat (a lesson we again failed to heed with mpox). We also need to understand and get comfortable with the difference between science and policy—for example, saying a vaccine or mask *mandate* won't be accepted or adhered to by the target audience from a policy standpoint isn't the same as saying vaccines or masks themselves are ineffective.

MISINFORMATION AND DISINFORMATION

While those of us in the doctors group were doing our best to clarify the health information underlying federal COVID-19 recommendations and policies, we were up against two other rapidly spreading pandemics: misinformation and disinformation. Misinformation is misleading information that's partially true or taken out of context but isn't intended to mislead. For example, someone saying you shouldn't get a COVID-19 vaccine because it "causes myocarditis." The mRNA vaccines *can* cause myocarditis in extremely rare cases. However, the chances of this happening are tiny, and nearly all cases of vaccine-induced myocarditis are mild, especially compared to the far greater chances of developing myocarditis from COVID-19. Leaving out those facts puts this unqualified statement about COVID-19 vaccines causing myocarditis in the category of misinformation. Disinformation is the spreading of intentionally false information. For example, consider "COVID-19 vaccines can change your DNA." The messenger RNA in COVID-19 vaccines never enters the cell nucleus, so it can't change or affect our DNA in any way,[106] yet many people will try to convince others of this fallacy to further an agenda. Disinformation peddlers will often encourage you to attend their seminars (for a fee) or buy unproven medications or supplements from them so they can make money.

The media identified the "Disinformation Dozen:" twelve individuals, including several doctors, who spread the majority of disinformation about COVID-19 on social media.[107] These folks positioned themselves as outsiders who would tell you the truth, contradicting the information coming from the government. Adopting simple narratives that match with our view of ourselves as bold, brave nonconformists can distort our understanding of complex, nuanced situations and even lead to tragic outcomes, yet these narratives can make us feel special and important. As we saw with the Disinformation Dozen, the story of "I'm a rebel and truth-teller who is looking out for you" can build a personal brand and create the opportunity to make a lot of money and gain a lot of attention and admiration.

Having professionals with expertise in communication advising public health officials could help us cut through a lot of the noise in the future, and we desperately need more research into how to best combat misinformation and disinformation!

As the current US surgeon general Vivek Murthy, who is a friend of mine, has said, misinformation and disinformation threaten US health and constitute a public health emergency. He wrote in his 2021 advisory on confronting misinformation, "Limiting the spread of health misinformation is a moral and civic imperative that will require a whole-of-society effort."[108]

It would also be helpful if television and film writers put more effort into collaborating with public health officials to develop storylines about health that could increase the amount of quality health information consumed by the public. We can often do more to spread health knowledge and influence public behavior via a *Law and Order* episode or with a well-placed nugget in the latest Netflix series than with an announcement from the surgeon general. I have to wonder if more people would have the latest COVID-19 vaccine booster if public health officials teamed more often with influencers, celebrities, Mad Men, and script writers who could artfully present the reasons we should be confident in the value of vaccines—a message we continue to have challenges communicating.

CHAPTER 10

VACCINE BREAKTHROUGH

SEEING HOSPITALS OVERWHELMED YET AGAIN throughout late summer and into the fall of 2020 was disturbing, but there was a bright light on the horizon: the development of vaccines was moving ahead far faster than anyone had predicted. Yet, given the rise in vaccine hesitancy predating the vaccine and increasingly heated rhetoric around our national COVID-19 response, it should have been no surprise that vaccines would soon become politicized.

In October, the first question at the vice presidential debates was about COVID-19. Then-senator Kamala Harris said the administration "covered up" that they knew the virus was "airborne" by January 28, citing Bob Woodward in his book *Rage*. As I said, some *suspected* the virus might be airborne as early as January, which is quite different from *knowing* it was airborne.[109] Lack of knowledge about transmission is why nearly everyone in public health, including the CDC and WHO, were saying as late as March that the general public didn't need to wear masks. Ironically, Woodward's book actually showed that neither President Trump nor Dr. Fauci used the word "airborne" during their discussions that week.[110] I get that Senator Harris may not have understood the difference between a virus being "airborne" and being carried in the air via droplets, but still, the politically motivated accusations were ill-informed or, at least, ill communicated, further increasing public confusion around the virus. (It's also noteworthy that while she was adamant during campaigning that Trump knew the virus was airborne yet kept it from the public, the Biden administration waited over a year from that debate statement—longer than it had been from January 28 to that debate—to finally and half-heartedly recommend high-filtration masks that could protect the public from an airborne virus.)

Senator Harris went on to say that she would trust Dr. Fauci and "public health professionals" if they were to recommend a vaccine, but she insisted that "If Donald Trump tells us we should take it, I'm not taking it." This statement reflected a gross (and dangerously misleading) misunderstanding of our vaccine approval system: We have a vigorous FDA approval process and a further CDC advisory committee on immunization practices to ensure no president can just "tell us to take" a vaccine. Implying otherwise was a direct attack on the integrity of the entire system—and vaccine hesitancy based largely on mistrust of that system already harms disproportionately high numbers of African Americans. Casting doubt on vaccine safety is a hard bell to un-ring. Despite the narratives, Senator Harris was actually the first and remains the highest ranked political figure of either party to say she might not trust a COVID-19 vaccine (New York Governor Andrew Cuomo was the second, saying, "Frankly, I'm not going to trust the federal government's opinion [on Covid vaccines], and I wouldn't recommend to New Yorkers based on the federal government's opinion."[111] This was many many months—and a presidential election—before Florida Governor

Ron DeSantis would be chastised for saying the exact same thing.) It was extremely frustrating to see someone who was vying to be the future vice president—and who would become the most prominent African American in the Biden administration—politicizing the vaccine. She in essence told people not to trust it unless Democrats won the election.

On December 18, 2020, Vice President Pence and I would get our vaccines in front of millions live on morning television, to help instill already flagging public confidence. I didn't want to be accused of "jumping the line," but the need to demonstrate that I as surgeon general believed the vaccines were safe—particularly to Black and Brown communities and especially in light of Harris's remarks—are a major part of why I decided to go ahead. To reassure and encourage the public, Whoopi Goldberg spoke on *The View* about getting vaccinated at New York City's Javits Center, telling viewers she couldn't even feel the shot,[112] and BET aired video of Tyler Perry receiving his vaccine and talking about Black Americans' understandable skepticism of the medical community.[113] I'm grateful to every public figure who worked to assure Americans that vaccines are an excellent investment in their health and the health of their communities.

I understand that it's difficult to both criticize an incumbent political opponent while encouraging people to trust systems and officials put in place by said opponent, but politicians have to do better. Governor DeSantis of Florida said in June 2022, "We are affirmatively against the COVID vaccine for young kids. These are the people who have *zero* risk of getting anything."[114] Such a statement certainly feels like disinformation as it's clearly untrue (children are at lower risk, but not at zero risk), and many feel it was made for political gain. By the end of 2021, COVID-19 had killed hundreds of US children, including over twenty in DeSantis's state of Florida. In fact, more kids died of COVID-19 in 2021 than 2020, making it a leading cause of death for people under eighteen.[115] Plus, his statement disregarded harms from long COVID, and from infected children passing the virus on to vulnerable adults at home or school. In my opinion, it's both appropriate and necessary to discuss the pros and cons of policy tradeoffs, yet we can't have legitimate discussion and debate when we dismiss harms that don't fit our narratives. Both "sides" have continually been guilty of this political obfuscation.

James Lawler, MD, an expert on Ebola and COVID-19, the director of International Programs and Innovation at the Global Center for Health Security, and hardly someone seen as being political, has said, "More lives have been lost during the Biden administration than the Trump administration, demonstrating there are institutional issues at play that go far beyond who is president."[116] I'd add that politics get in the way too, because people let their loyalty to the "home team" influence how they view situations more than the health information and science.

Some on the Left repeated Biden's oft stated line that COVID-19 was a "pandemic of the unvaccinated," largely so as to cast blame on red states and conservatives. This public shaming didn't exactly inspire the unvaccinated to hurry to get a shot. The narrative served a political purpose, but in the interests of public health, we must look at the full array of who fails to take protective measures and why. COVID-19 exposed a problem we had known about for years: vaccine hesitancy, which has more than one cause. Sometimes, the problems are practical. Some people intend to get vaccinated but they may not have transportation or might be focused on more immediately pressing health issues. Some may be leery of experiencing vaccine side effects that will force them miss work. (Companies can support vaccinations by providing paid time off for their employees to get vaccinated and to have time off to recover, if needed.)

Also, many people don't appreciate the importance of vaccine boosters. We were fortunate that our vaccines were highly effective, more so than we expected. However, they are not as durable as we had hoped. In other words, you need to be vaccinated more than once to be optimally protected against future infection. People need to know that until we develop even better vaccines, boosters will remain crucial tools for preventing hospitalization and death. You can get the annual flu vaccine and a COVID-19 booster on the same day or get one and then the other, but please don't delay because you believe they're not important or because you think they have to be 100 percent effective at preventing infection and sickness to have value. Remember: layers of protection should be your aim, so get your vaccines according to the CDC recommendations.

Another contributor to vaccine hesitancy is misinformation about the risks of vaccines versus the risks of contracting the illness or disease. Many people don't understand that the risk of vaccine related side effects or health problems are far smaller for most people than the health risks of the disease. Often, people tell themselves, "Well, my chances of dying from COVID-19 are very low," but low risk isn't "no" risk. Further, risk extends to more than just death (the truth is the majority of people infected with most any vaccine preventable disease actually survive their infection). COVID-19 vaccines not only reduce risk of hospitalization and death; they reduce the risk of long COVID-19 by as much as 29 percent.[117] And long COVID-19 continues to affect many: 2.5 percent of those who have symptomatic COVID-19 experience symptoms for three months or longer while 60 percent of those hospitalized with COVID-19 are still experiencing long COVID-19 six months later.[118] You might survive an acute infection only to suffer or even eventually die from long COVID-19.[119] Yes, we have treatments for COVID-19, but not all of them work for everyone, and the virus mutates around them. For example, monoclonal antibodies are no longer effective for COVID-19 treatment.[120] Prevention will always be better than a cure.

It would also be helpful if people could more easily access a primary care provider who knows their health history and with whom they can have frank discussions about health risks. Many people (especially younger adults) don't visit a doctor unless they're sick, so they don't have someone they can ask about vaccines or preventable health risks. And people lacking health insurance (more common in "red" states) rarely have a relationship with a medical professional who can debunk the misinformation and disinformation they encounter.

Also, doctors and nurses need to communicate better, and make sure people feel heard. A friend of mine had healthcare power of attorney for her mother, who was in hospice care in the end stages of pulmonary fibrosis. One day, a hospice nurse called to tell her that her mother had slipped into a coma for no apparent reason. My friend later learned that her mother had been given a flu vaccine without her official permission. When her mother passed a day later, my friend asked the nurse practitioner whether this would be reported to some medical authority as it might at least contribute to important data that would guide doctors in treating patients like her mom. He said the event was purely coincidental, so he wouldn't report it. She didn't know that she could have done so. Even in the likely event that these events were in fact unrelated, these types of incidents cause people to mistrust the medical community. We need to help people feel they are not being lectured at, talked down to, or dismissed. If you feel that way as a patient, don't hesitate to change physicians or nurse practitioners.

OPERATION WARP SPEED

Named after the phenomenon in *Star Trek* where the starship suddenly shifts into the fastest possible speed, Operation Warp Speed was a federal collaboration between government agencies and pharmaceutical companies in a race to create and distribute COVID-19 vaccines and therapeutics. The doctors on the White House Coronavirus Task Force were mostly excluded from the project, which from a federal perspective was viewed as more of a logistical and financial enterprise than a scientific one. (The scientific development would be left largely to the private companies, with the exception of the NIH and Moderna collaboration.) I am, however, quite proud of my own efforts to help promote diversity in the pool of subjects in the clinical trials after NIH director Francis Collins highlighted how few minorities were participating. Especially on the heels of largely Democratic skepticism at the time about the speed of vaccine development, it truly would have been a disaster for vaccine trust in Black and

Brown communities if minority enrollment had remained in the single-digit percentages as it was in August of 2020. That's when Dr. Collins, Dr. Fauci, and I started meeting with pharmaceutical companies every Saturday morning to figure out how to increase enrollment of people of color in their studies. Between August 2020 and late November of that year, diversity in the COVID-19 trials increased to over 30 percent. It's one of the more remarkable and least talked about aspects of COVID-19 vaccine development, and it has led to a complete change in the way the FDA and pharmaceutical and device industries consider the importance (and feasibility) of diversity in clinical trials.

One aim of Operation Warp Speed was to remove any financial risks that might disincentivize companies from developing a vaccine as quickly as possible. Federal dollars were used to pre-purchase vaccines and secure or build facilities where vaccines could be mass produced. While the project didn't cut corners it did cut regulatory red tape, allowing for overlapping phases of drug development. This saved many months (or years) in the process. Additionally, drug company researchers were able to continuously dispatch data to the FDA and receive real-time feedback to facilitate much faster authorization once all the data was in. Unfortunately, financing for COVID-19 vaccine research has been continually and significantly cut in recent years, so while other countries are already working towards developing newer nasal-spray COVID-19 vaccines, we're unlikely to see anything like this in the US for some time. Alternative vaccines could increase the breadth and durability of our immunity as well as help address some of the reasons for vaccine hesitancy, but without the federal will and funding to power our development engines, our ability to travel at "warp speed" has been severely compromised.

Operation Warp Speed fulfilled its mission to deliver vaccines, but vaccines aren't the same as vaccinations. Between rising vaccine hesitancy pre-pandemic, politicization, and public unawareness about mRNA technology, many worried that the vaccines weren't safe and effective. Disinformation and misinformation continues to abound. Further, initially, the Trump administration—and then the Biden administration—defined "effective" largely in terms of stopping disease transmission. Such statements have become increasingly problematic as we now know the vaccines now only prevent infection for about three to four months.

Leaders in public health need to work on messaging about the safety and effectiveness of vaccines and help people understand why, when, and for whom boosters are needed. Because the COVID-19 vaccines turned out to be less durable than we had hoped, many believed public health officials were lying about their effectiveness. The truth however is that current vaccines and boosters are still highly effective at preventing hospitalization and death, and they're as durable as the flu shot has ever been.

Also, while some referred to mRNA vaccine technology as "new," researchers had been developing it for over a decade— we just hadn't needed to deploy this technology in a pandemic yet. To adapt it for SARSCoV2 we only had to switch out the genetic code, like taking out the old game cartridge from your PlayStation and inserting a new one. So, once Pfizer, Moderna, and others were provided with the financial fuel and regulatory assistance they needed, the race to warp speed was on. By

December 2020, the first COVID-19 vaccines were available to people not participating in clinical trials.[121] Given the glacial pace of subsequent vaccine authorization for children, final vaccine approval for adults, and authorization and roll out of boosters, it's hard to downplay the historic and lifesaving accomplishments of OWS, or to argue progress would've occurred as quickly under different leadership.

WHO SHOULD BE FIRST IN LINE?

As with testing, vaccine access posed not just logistical but ethical challenges. Who should be at the front of the line and why? To make a point about priorities, a critical care nurse in New York City named Sandra Lindsay, who had immigrated from Jamaica, was chosen to be the first person outside of a clinical trial to be vaccinated. (I had the opportunity to meet Sandra, and she is both a lovely and a brave person, as were the thousands of people who participated in vaccine trials so we could feel and be safe getting vaccinated for COVID.) The agreed upon plan was to first make vaccines available to healthcare workers, after that, to nursing home patients, and then to essential workers who didn't work in healthcare, especially those in communities deemed at higher risk.[122]

In retrospect, the recommendations could have been more specific about individual risk, but to be honest, everyone was caught a little off guard by the speed with which the vaccines were ready for public consumption, and DC was a little distracted by this "small" election that was happening. A lesson is that *future crisis response plans need to include professional ethics committees to discuss and communicate the pros and cons of allocation strategies for limited resources, and we need to involve them before and not after the resources are available.*

People very loosely described as healthcare workers who were not exactly at risk for encountering sick COVID-19 patients (psychologists doing telehealth visits, for example, or young and healthy dental hygienists employed by dental offices that still remained shut down) were able to go to the front of the line and often did so unapologetically. In a vaccine "Hunger Games," that was looked at as a ticket to normalcy, many were vaccinated far ahead of others who were clearly at higher risk. *In the future, we need to do a better job collecting demographic data related to risk and helping people understand why certain groups should be prioritized.* At a micro-level, a grocery worker or car service driver who also was from a marginalized community and/or caring for an elderly family member had a greater argument for a vaccine than a middle-class receptionist at a surgery center who was getting paid to stay home because the facility was shut down, or who had the privilege of teleworking. At a macro-level, we should have anticipated that overly broad guidelines would be taken advantage of by those at lower risk, while others at higher risk would be left on the outside looking in. One result was grumbling from people who didn't understand the decision-making process and felt it wasn't fair. Another was even worse: some people were unduly harmed (often while providing services for the rest of us) because they weren't afforded the opportunity to protect themselves.

When explaining health equity, I often give the example of a person needing a wheelchair. The federal government doesn't provide wheelchairs to everyone, just people who actually need them. Not everyone needs a ramp to enter a public building, but some do so we spend extra money to make it accessible. We're not discriminating against people who feel they have an equal "right" to a wheelchair or a ramp because they would *prefer* to have such things; we're ensuring accessibility to people who truly *need* it. In an effort to distribute vaccines as quickly as possible, we failed to do it as equitably as possible. We relied on people recognizing that while, technically speaking, they fit into a certain priority group, in actuality, they could actually be hurting others who were at higher risk by consuming limited resources. Similarly, we saw that the false belief that hydroxychloroquine can prevent or treat COVID-19 created shortages of the medication for those who actually needed it. The run on hydroxychloroquine was highly problematic for lupus patients who take it regularly.[123] Wants versus needs can play out in ugly and harmful ways, especially when limited supply and high demand meet a lack of clear and accurate information.

The equitable and efficient distribution of vaccines was also complicated by regional issues. As with ventilators and PPE, many of the distribution decisions were occurring at the state and local level. Without a real-time data dashboard to understand who was putting vaccines in arms (and who had vaccines expiring on shelves), it was hard to assist with fair allocation. Fortunately, things moved so quickly that it actually wasn't that long before most adults who wanted a vaccine could get one. In fact, we got to that point well before Dr. Fauci and other experts had previously predicted we'd even have a vaccine. Despite largely political claims of a "botched" rollout, this was the largest and fastest distribution of vaccines in history, and it went about as well in the US as it did in most other countries. We also never would have even had the luxury of discussing distribution if the Trump administration hadn't exceeded everyone's wildest expectations with Operation Warp Speed. Even so, *we need to do a better job next time to proactively ensure not just speed but also fairness and equity in distributing limited resources, including new vaccines and treatments.*

THE MANDATE QUESTION

Should vaccines have been mandated? What about masks? I'm often asked these questions by the media, at talks, and by family and friends. From a scientific standpoint, the evidence is clear that mandates have historically been an extremely valuable public health tool. Further, vaccine requirements have always been a topic of debate, but mandates to promote national health and security have a long-established precedent (going all the way back to George Washington).[124] For instance, we've long accepted that if you work in a hospital, you must maintain certain vaccinations to protect patients. The military and public schools also require vaccinations to protect not just individuals but institutions.

Misinformation about COVID-19 vaccines being required for kids to attend school went viral in November 2022, which gave me an opportunity to help the public understand something about vaccinations. Most vaccines that have traditionally been mandated are also ones that have been widely accepted as durable and safe, but lowering the *individual* risk of harm isn't actually the goal of most mandates. This is important to understand, because so much of the debate over mandates has been focused on the extremely high survivability of a COVID-19 infection, especially in young people. Yet, children get vaccinated against measles despite the minimal chance that any particular child will suffer serious acute or long-term harm (for example, blindness) if they contract the virus. As a society, we accept this mandate because of the largely preventable disruption to our daily lives that outbreaks can cause and because the vaccine provides our children with long-term protection against what can occasionally be a debilitating or even deadly disease. Of course, a small chance of harm multiplied by a large number of people still equals significant morbidity and mortality, and if it ends up being *your* child disabled or killed by a disease for which they are unvaccinated, the risk of harm becomes 100 percent.

Recognizing the difference between durable and non-durable vaccines, only a handful of states require flu vaccines for kids, and even then, they're only for kids in pre-K or childcare.[125] COVID-19 vaccines were added to the CDC's recommended schedule of childhood vaccines not to facilitate mandates but to allow parents more choice through the Vaccines for Children (VFC) program. However, given the low durability of current COVID-19 vaccines, it's very unlikely that being on the schedule will lead to them being required for children to attend school in your state. In addition, no state has mandated any vaccine for school attendance while it is under Emergency Use Authorization, and I don't expect (and wouldn't support) COVID-19 vaccines as the exception. Even the laws contemplated or passed in states like California specifically stated that they will not take effect unless and until the vaccines are fully approved.

Another important point to this conversation about mandates is that not all unvaccinated people are "anti-vaxxers" who must be compelled to do the right thing. Many are vaccine-hesitant, meaning they can be persuaded to vaccinate through education and building of trust, or by addressing pragmatic barriers to getting vaccinated. I also believe we need to better understand and accommodate legitimate medical concerns about vaccines without allowing personal exemptions from longstanding vaccine mandates for dubious reasons, such as simply being philosophically opposed. Of course, it's hard to make any policy for millions of people without some abuse of the rules and without at least a few people unfairly left out, but we could more carefully consider how strict or loose those rules are. In some states, it has become too easy to claim a philosophical or questionable religious objection (or even make up a religion) to get out of having your kids vaccinated. This gaming of the system simply isn't fair to society. Again, vaccine mandates are *not* about protecting an individual but about protecting the *public* from the individual.

Overall, I firmly believe the best way to encourage and increase vaccination is by building relationships and educating people about vaccine safety and efficacy. That's why *we need trusted and local health advocates explaining vaccine safety and the unique benefits and risks of vaccinations.*

Having vaccinations easily available at drugstores or mass vaccination sites is good—especially when there is urgency. However, ideally, people will have a relationship with a healthcare provider who can answer questions and help address reasons for vaccine hesitancy. One problem with the mass vaccination infrastructure of the pandemic is that it didn't always allow for a one-on-one conversation with a trusted health provider. That meant if someone was unsure, they just didn't get show up to get vaccinated.

In my opinion, when we are contemplating mandates, we must work to ensure public comprehension and trust are at high levels *before* the mandate. Ironically, the people in your target audience need to already believe in the value of vaccination for societal buy-in for mandates to occur. For example, most people whose children are unvaccinated against measles aren't against the *idea* of the vaccine. They understand why mandates are in place, and their kids are vaccinated against other diseases, but these parents are either mildly hesitant or complacent. Regardless, a mandate in that instance can give them a nudge to visit their health provider. True "anti-vaxxers" aren't going to get their kids vaccinated no matter what you say or do, but they gain more people to their side when those who are merely vaccine-hesitant are demonized simply for asking questions. In other words, mandates get you from the herd immunity five-yard line to the end zone, but they aren't effective as a "Hail Mary" pass from sixty yards of mistrust away.

Also, policymakers should consider this: if you're requiring masking, testing, and vaccines, will all of these be free *and* easily available to everyone regardless of their socioeconomic status? One of the problems with our "sick care" system is that even when we say a medical item or procedure is "free," that's not always truly the case. Unexpected bills have burned too many Americans: for example, a "free" annual screening for breast cancer can get a diagnostic code added to it if the X-ray shows an anomaly and more images are taken. A "free" annual physical suddenly might cost extra because the patient brought up a concern that justifies the addition of a consultation code. A screening colonoscopy is free, but if a polyp is found and removed, insurance might deny payment or require a copay. While the Affordable Care Act was instrumental in making it much easier for millions of people to get preventive care and all vaccines are technically covered 100 percent by health insurance, Medicaid, and Medicare, I'd like to see the ACA updated to address some of these problems. I'd also like to see a massive communications campaign to help more people understand their benefits and rights. Bad or poorly explained or enforced policies and hidden costs have caused too many Americans to lose trust in the medical community.

Mandates often come up because employers have a further and compelling interest in maintaining safe spaces for customers and employees and likewise in schools for students and staff. However, they can accomplish this goal by offering options: for example, make it as easy as possible for people to get vaccinated with on-site clinics and time off to get vaccines. If one still chooses not to get vaccinated, it may make sense to ask them to wear a mask at all times, or submit to testing, or work or attend class from home to keep others safe. Such precautions are especially important during an uptick in cases. There is often more than one way (beyond mandates) to maintain safety in a workplace or school setting.

Also, those of us in public health must remember that giving people agency makes sense from a behavioral standpoint. If you tell them they must comply with only one course of action, many will rebel at the lack of choice. That's especially true when the one choice you're offering is shown not to be as highly effective as originally thought, as has been the case for vaccines, mask wearing, *and* social distancing. Whenever feasible, let people choose the layers that work best for them.

Of course, and again, one of the reasons we have so much vaccine hesitancy is misinformation and disinformation. Another is how we speak to each other: whether we listen well and express empathy *before* offering a rebuttal, or worse, an insult. It's vitally important to choose our words carefully and not let anger or contempt—or politics—choose them for us. Even the best communicators can benefit from reflecting on whether their way of communicating is serving or hindering the goal of health. We need to have conversations about COVID-19 and other health issues so we can protect ourselves, our families, and our communities.

• CHAPTER 11 •

WEATHERING THE STORM

ON TUESDAY, NOVEMBER 3, 2020, in the highest voter turnout since 1900, the American people chose Joe Biden as their next president. In part due to fears of contracting COVID-19 and in part due to fear of four more years of Trump, historically high numbers of Americans, particularly Democrats and Left-leaning Independents, cast absentee votes. Also, some election workers (who tend to be seniors and therefore at higher risk for COVID-19 complications) chose to stay home as they had for most of 2020, fearing infection. Knowing this might happen caused many to anticipate long lines.[126] Anyone following the news recognized the likelihood of Trump looking like the winner *initially*, only to have his lead reduced as more votes were counted. In a very real sense, long simmering debates about voting methods and vote counting came to a boil because of the virus. Twenty years after the infamous Bush versus Gore election, COVID-19 became 2020's "hanging chad." As the hours passed on election day, rumors of issues at the polls ran rampant, and political disinformation machines were in high gear. Pundits, politicians, and media personalities would boost their brands with claims of massive voter fraud—especially pertaining to absentee ballots.

Once it was clear Biden had actually won, I was determined for the sake of the American people to do whatever I could to provide a smooth transition. I prioritized connecting with Dr. Vivek Murthy. (Despite being appointed by different presidents and political parties, the former surgeons general are a small and close group.) Dr. Murthy had spoken at the Democratic National Committee's nominating convention in support of then-presidential candidate Joe Biden. It's worth noting that no prior "Nation's Doctor" had ever weighed in at a party nominating convention or been featured so publicly as part of a partisan political campaign, so this was historically unprecedented. President-elect Biden had already stated Dr. Murthy would be "his" surgeon general—though I still had a year left on my term in the role. (The role of surgeon general is a presidential appointment, but it is also technically for a four-year term.)

Historically, many surgeons general have finished their terms across administrations. In recent times as health has become more politicized, that has been the case less and less. Dr. Murthy himself was asked to resign from his first term after serving several months in the Trump administration. This was a move Democrats, including prominent Senate Health Committee member Chris Murphy of Connecticut, criticized harshly at the time. In the words of Senator Murphy, "Surgeons general are not supposed to be fired mid-term. They have served administrations of both political parties because keeping Americans safe and healthy isn't a partisan issue. By firing Dr. Murthy, President Trump is politicizing the position of surgeon general and risking the credibility of our nation's top public health official."[127]

I congratulated my friend Dr. Murthy and told him I would be happy to stay on until he was nominated and confirmed. The process can take months (and during his first tenure, it took over a year). I even offered to reach out to Republican senators to help with his confirmation. I told him I would gladly step down as soon as he could assume the role and I would publicly state my intentions of doing so. For the sake of our country, I wanted a smooth transition, even if the new administration wanted a different person in the role. Dr. Murthy told me he would speak to the Biden transition team but that this plan made sense and he supported it.[128] After all, the Trump administration allowed him to stay on for several months after inauguration to create a smooth transition—and that wasn't even in the midst of a once-in-a-century health crisis.

Typically, when a new administration takes office, they sweep out the door most political appointees, including major health officials like the heads of the FDA, the CMS, and the CDC. There's no reason a new president shouldn't be able to pick their own administrators and agency heads, especially when those folks will be responsible for helping execute stated administration goals that helped said president get elected. But when there's an ongoing public health emergency, stable leadership (or any leadership) and a smooth transition is clearly in the public's best interest. Infection rates were rising as temperatures were falling, and people were spending more time indoors. Plus, we were still expecting increased travel and gatherings—and infections—related to the Thanksgiving and Christmas holidays, not to mention the massive public gatherings in celebration of Biden's election that were taking place in cities across America. (The celebrations I witnessed in DC after the 2020 election were as packed, and nearly as maskless, as any Trump event I'd been to since the start of the pandemic—and again this was still pre-vaccine).

Despite my misguided belief that just as Dr. Murthy had stayed on for a bit with the Trump administration, I would be doing the same with Biden's, the day before the inauguration, I received a voicemail from a junior-level staffer coldly asking when the transition team could "expect to receive my resignation." Apparently, my offer to stay on until Dr. Murthy was confirmed had been rejected—though no one had bothered to tell me until mere hours before the transition began. President Biden chose to dismiss the entire White House Coronavirus Task Force at a critical time in the pandemic. I believe this decision cost time and lives and was purely political. (It would've cost the administration nothing to keep the current team on as advisors for a few weeks—and all were willing. But it didn't fit the political narrative that anyone Trump had appointed wasn't just useless, but dangerous.) Increasing vaccine access was paramount, the virus was mutating again, and we were just starting to learn about long-term COVID-19 symptoms.[129],[130] The only person retained was Dr. Fauci, who, as stated earlier, was viewed by the public and media as being anti-Trump and was felt by many to be a Democrat and Biden supporter. He was also appointed to be Biden's "special medical advisor," something Biden had announced as far back as June 2020 and highlighted throughout his campaign.[131] Though I have and will continue to criticize the horrific and unfair treatment of Dr. Fauci and his service, I believe this was a key turning point in the public's perception of him. Instantly, he went from being viewed mostly as a career government servant—an apolitical NIAID director who had served seven presidents in that capacity—to a handpicked "special advisor" to Joe Biden and, in essence, a (Democratic) political appointee. Further and whether he liked it or not, Fauci became a major Biden campaign surrogate. "A vote for Biden is a vote for Fauci," became a rallying cry of the Democratic party. Ironically, the political independence and governmental separation that had made Dr. Fauci distinct from the other doctors on the task force in the Trump administration was now turned on its head. As a Biden-appointee and the one person on the original COVID-19 task force openly spoken about at campaign events (of both parties), he became a clear target of those objecting to the Biden administration.

The administration did keep on General Gustave Perna and Moncef Slaoui, the two professionals most responsible for developing and implementing the vaccine plan. I'd had a good working relationship with both men but interacted far more with General Perna, who oversaw the logistics of mass production and distribution of the vaccines. We shared a degree of respect and connection because we both wore the uniform—I was a three-star admiral, and he was a four-star general. Also, he was clearly concerned about diversity and health equity, which I appreciated. General Perna reached out to me often and involved me in meetings where he felt my perspectives on inclusion would be valuable, even when other officials in the administration didn't feel my input was necessary. He came to me for assistance when we needed outreach to minority communities and historically Black colleges and universities (HBCUs) to ensure equitable distribution of resources and buy-in for vaccines. I made calls and assembled college and university presidents and community leaders at his request. I firmly believe this would not have happened unless someone like me, an African American physician who already had relationships with these groups, was at the table. It also wouldn't have happened without the support of General Perna.

The Biden administration's first and loudest complaint was that there was no national vaccine production or distribution plan. I felt this was completely unfair and unfounded, as it dismissed the hard work of everyone on Operation Warp Speed, including hundreds of career public servants and private industry partners who sacrificed much to deliver a vaccine faster than anyone thought possible. President Biden also said the Trump administration had not provided important information regarding COVID-19.[132] While others, including Alyssa Farah Griffin, the former White House director of strategic communications, have asserted that to be the case from some inside the White House, my personal experience was that everyone at HHS was working hard to ensure a smooth transition. Unfortunately, they were meeting political obstacles from both sides of the aisle.[133]

When it comes to health, and especially in a crisis, people die when there isn't a smooth changeover. Hospital safety protocols focus on changeovers between shifts of nurses and doctors as critical points at which inefficiencies occur and errors are often made. *Incoming and outgoing leaders need to put people over politics and make a point of acknowledging, thanking (instead of denigrating), and working with apolitical public servants of previous administrations.* This would reassure Americans that everyone is working toward a smooth transition, and protecting the health of the citizenry. And it would save lives.

With my job winding down, my wife and kids moved back to Indiana. At one point (somewhat comically), I had trouble securing a mortgage on my new home because the mortgage company needed written proof of former employment, and the new administration wouldn't verify that I had once been the US surgeon general. (This moment went viral when I jokingly tweeted about it, and it was covered by several news outlets.)[134] I needed to stay in DC because I had to continue working clinically at Walter Reed Hospital to keep my medical license active and to maintain health insurance for my family for a few more weeks. Back I went to living in my friend's garage apartment. I tell you this not to make you feel sorry for me, but so you understand what many people—most without the means and savings of an anesthesiologist—can go through when they commit to public service. This scenario is especially common with political appointees: the appointments often start and end abruptly. It makes it difficult for those with families to serve and nearly impossible for people without significant wealth or savings to make such a commitment. It's one underappreciated reason why we often end up with only a select viewpoint in decision-making rooms: White, wealthy, older, empty nesters.

JANUARY 6

Leading up to Inauguration Day, there was a flurry of activity to facilitate departure and transition. Some of it was professional and legally required, such as receiving security debriefings and making sure we properly saved and turned over federal records.

Some was personal, for example, sharing contact information and planning goodbye meetings with those with whom you'd been in the "foxhole" over the past few stressful years. There was also a planned "rally" scheduled for January 6 for people to express their support of President Trump and their belief that the election results were invalid. At the time, this meant little more to me than it did to any other average citizen watching the political hullabaloo that was going on. I believed that despite the rhetoric from both Trump and the media, power would be handed over peacefully on Inauguration Day, as it had between presidents for over two centuries. People forget that Hillary Clinton cast doubt on the validity of 2016 election results, even saying, Trump "knows he's an illegitimate president… I know that he knows this wasn't on the level."[135] But there was still a peaceful transition of power after that election.

On January 5, 2021, HHS notified employees that protests were expected near the Capitol building and that federal workers with offices nearby were advised to work from home. Washington, DC, is protest central, especially in the area where I worked (within view and earshot of the Capitol and the Supreme Court). Since 2017, I'd received countless such warnings that hadn't led to any significant problems. Knowing that the Secret Service guarded the secretary of HHS and would be in the building, I felt safe going to my office that day. The day before, I had no problems getting to and from the White House for our final task force meeting (which Vice President Pence led but President Trump didn't attend).

When I peered out my office window on the morning of January 6, it seemed that the rally seemed to be shaping up as a big nothing burger near the Capitol. A few people with MAGA hats or Trump flags were milling around, but there was little more foot traffic than on a typical day on the mall. I turned on the TV in my office and saw the activity at the White House. It resembled what I had witnessed while traveling with the president in his motorcade: fans cheering, smiling, and waving flags. It was indeed a rally-like atmosphere, complete with the Village People's "YMCA" playing in the background. I bet my office staff that the president would do his awkward shimmy dance to pump up the crowd, and of course he did. Once he finished speaking from the White House, I turned off my television and went back to work.

As I sat in my office, I occasionally glanced out the window. The crowd in front of the Capitol slowly began to build, chanting and even dancing. After an hour or so, I realized the sounds of the crowd were taking on a different, more energetic tone—perhaps even an ominous one. Maybe it was time for me to leave?

I decided to head over to Secretary Azar's office to see if he had any concerns about the growing (and increasingly agitated) crowd and if he was planning to shut down the building. I also wanted to know if the Secret Service thought I'd have any problems departing and driving back to my apartment. A member of Secretary Azar's Secret Service detail told me that there had been bomb threats. Secretary Azar and I went to the top floor and out on a building balcony to get a better look at what was happening. Looking out at the Capitol, my first thought was, *Well, that's interesting. Speaker Pelosi is letting people onto her private balcony?* Then, Secretary Azar said, "The damned fools unfurled a [MAGA] flag from the Capitol roof!" Finally, it dawned on me that these visitors to the Speaker's office were not there by invitation.

We all went back downstairs, turned on the TV, and learned that the vice president was seemingly barricaded in the Capitol.

The entire scenario was surreal.

Was what I could see from HHS the work of a few rogue characters, or was something bigger afoot? Was the vice president—someone who had repeatedly supported me—in real danger? Should I be worried about the building I was in being blown up? I didn't want to get stuck in the office overnight if a curfew was imposed. Secretary Azar had said it wasn't his call, the Office of Personnel Management determined the opening and closing of federal buildings, and so far, no such announcement had come. Then, Secretary Azar muttered, "Screw this!" and announced to everyone that he wasn't waiting any longer. He was shutting down the building so we could get home safely. The mayor of DC would later declare a 6:00 p.m. curfew, but the decisive leadership that impacted my life that day was from Secretary Azar, not the White House or local DC leaders. While this may seem unrelated to my story about the pandemic, *it again shows the difficulty we continually run into when a crisis occurs and it's unclear who is in charge.* That lack of clarity and decisiveness didn't cost any lives at HHS that day, but it could have.

Though it may seem petty on the surface, before leaving HHS, my thoughts surprisingly turned to my wardrobe. You can never wear an admiral's uniform in public and not be noticed, but I figured a pro-Trump crowd was also likely to be pro-military. Surely, they wouldn't attack someone in uniform. (I would later discover how very wrong I was on that account. The brutality against officers that day was astonishing.) I certainly didn't want to be a Black man in civilian clothes walking amongst an agitated crowd where some people were proudly displaying Confederate flags. Knowing my life might be at risk if I made the wrong decision, I weighed my choices carefully. I finally decided to wear my uniform. The upside of being seen as a high-ranking military officer seemed greater than the downside of being recognized as part of the government (amongst a crowd in a decidedly anti-government mood). Though I also still chafe at being labeled "Trump's surgeon general," I figured if I ran into trouble that day, it would be a suitable time to immediately and loudly identify myself as such. Yet another lesson that is repeated throughout this book again was apparent on this fateful day: I couldn't make my decision without accounting for the facts that I was 1) a Black man; 2) likely to face more scrutiny than others for reasons beyond my control; and 3) inextricably associated with Trump.

In retrospect, I was unsafe either way, which I learned as I left for home. People were spilling over from the mall into the streets, so I drove with extreme caution. I didn't see any police officers helping to clear the crowd, so I inched forward carefully as agitated people yelling protest slogans crossed my path, walking down the middle of the street. Now was definitely not the time to give anyone a reason to attack my car, smash my windshield, accuse me of accidentally bumping them, or even notice me. It took an hour to go two blocks and get on the highway. I was never so glad to get back to my little garage apartment!

My life had been in full upheaval before, but in the days that followed (before I officially left my office for good on January 21), Washington, DC, became a drastically different place.

It transformed into a militarized zone with chain link fences, barbed wire, and armed soldiers everywhere. I needed special permission to enter HHS headquarters and had to go through multiple checkpoints to get there. The few times I went in, I was completely alone.

My feeling of isolation lifted when I connected with Chef José Andrés, with whom I'd first become acquainted when he was bashing me on Twitter. He was cooking meals for the National Guard troops in DC. Despite being in a city with some of the nicest hotel rooms in the world (almost all of which were sitting empty at the time), troops were actually sleeping in parking garages and eating MREs as if they were out in the middle of the Afghanistan desert. It bothered me to know that yet again, first responders were suffering from a lack of resources to support their mission, and yet again, the resources they needed were literally all around them!

I wanted to help in any way I could. I come from a military family and found it disgusting to see people in uniform treated that way. I was glad Chef José, who had made it clear he loathed Donald Trump, did not hold my position in Trump's administration against me. I eagerly joined him in passing out meals to National Guard members. They were grateful, but I was too. I was able to leave DC and move back home feeling glad that I'd been able to work "across the aisle" and do something tangible, however small, to help our nation recover from the ugly and painful events of January 6.

The actions of those who stormed the Capitol on January 6 had nearly toppled our government and with it, harmed our efforts to keep citizens safe from the pandemic. After that day, work on the pandemic transition from Trump's team to Biden's ground almost to a halt. From my perspective, it wasn't because people in HHS weren't committed to a smooth transition. It was because it's hard to work on such a transition when armed soldiers deny you access to your office, computer, and records. Trump and the politics surrounding him impacted our transition, but not only in the ways most people think.

On January 21, at the insistence of the Biden administration, I officially sent in my resignation, and an acting surgeon general took over: Rear Admiral Susan Orsega. While I highly respect Admiral Orsega, I was disappointed that the Biden administration passed over Rear Admiral Erica Schwartz—a decades-long career public servant (like Dr. Fauci) and the highest-ranking African American in HHS besides me. Unfortunately, she was connected to me: she had graciously agreed to leave her position as chief medical officer of the US Coast Guard early to serve as my deputy surgeon general. Of course, I was connected to Trump, and she was connected to me, so there's no way she could serve as surgeon general, even in an "acting" capacity.

THE PRICE OF SERVING

As the Nation's Doctor and as a human being, I fully admit I made my share of mistakes during my tenure. I'd do lots of things differently if I had another chance (who among us wouldn't?). However, I also know I did a lot to protect the health of the American people, and especially in marginalized communities and communities of color. Being only the second US surgeon general to have been a state health commissioner (thereby having critical relationships with others in that role) strongly impacted our federal ability to communicate effectively with states in a crisis and help them get what they needed to protect their citizens. As only the second Black US surgeon general, I shouldered the burden of being the sole representative of millions of Americans who too often don't have a voice in "the room where it happens." Coming from a rural community, I was often the only one at the table who knew what it was like when the city or suburban folks are making policies based on their life experiences, but your upbringing, values, and resources are vastly different. As a practicing physician, I fought for the clinicians who must implement and bear the risk of policies made by people who've never treated a patient (or at least not recently).

I'm proud of my contributions, but I'm also still processing the fact that I paid a high price personally and professionally for my missteps *and* my public service. For one thing, I've not received the traditional accolades, honorary degrees, awards, and opportunities common for a former US surgeon general. For example, in 2020, the National Academy of Medicine admitted a record number of new members, and their announced focus was on diversity. Many of those brought in were minorities and people committed to health equity and inclusion—things I've not only spent my life fighting for, but literally and visually symbolized. When I was first nominated for the Academy in 2019, I was informed that the Academy decided they shouldn't allow current political appointees to become members. Yet in 2021, multiple newly minted members of the Biden administration were admitted (though yet again, I wasn't and neither was anyone from the prior administration, including anyone affiliated with Operation Warp Speed, the greatest global health achievement of the last seventy-five years.)[136] Was all of this an objective reflection of my service as just the second African American male to serve as the surgeon general? Was my bipartisan work to advance harm reduction, both as state health commissioner where I helped expand syringe service programs across rural and conservative America and US surgeon general, via an historic naloxone advisory, taken into account? Was my omission coincidence? Was it something else? I'll let you decide. But the perception among many is that an inordinate number of supposedly non-political institutions preferentially include and favor loud-and-proud supporters of one political party while also seeming to exclude anyone who is thought of as too conservative. This seems to be the case despite comparable qualifications and is especially true if the potential member has any affiliation with Trump. The lesson is this: *many health and medical organizations and institutions risk becoming political echo chambers, appearing to be both passively and actively biased against conservatives even as they often lament that they don't know how to get through to conservative America.* (After science magazine *Nature* published their endorsement of Biden, a study showed many conservatives viewed them as less credible than previously, which is another example of the cost of politicizing health and science.)[137]

No well-compensated Fortune 500 board positions were forthcoming for me either. This may seem inconsequential or petty to bring up, but Black men are underrepresented in terms of such opportunities (as well for as the accolades I mentioned). So, it's noteworthy that even one of the most accomplished Black male physicians in US history has had trouble breaking through the glass ceiling—although perhaps this is because of some very non-traditional sources of discrimination for someone who looks like me.

Also, in a financial sense, I paid—literally—for the privilege of my public service. I took a 60 percent pay cut from what I earned as a practicing anesthesiologist. "Hey, you still made more as surgeon general than most Americans do!" is a frequent refrain when I bring up this financial hit. But how many of you parents, homeowners, and/or single income families could—or voluntarily would—withstand an abrupt 60 percent decrease in your monthly income only to be badgered and belittled and even to receive death threats for your efforts?

I'd worked hard to save for my retirement early in my career. African Americans, even highly educated ones, statistically lag far behind their white counterparts in retirement savings and wealth accumulation, in part because of the sense that helping one's family and community financially has to be a top priority. I was determined to be different, but once my pay decreased, Lacey and I had to significantly dip into our life savings to pay for our move and to live in the costly DMV area.

To relocate, we'd had to sell our "forever" home in Indiana, something my wife still hasn't forgiven me for. We'd had no choice but to sell low and buy high in a tumultuous time for real estate, and when buying our new house in Indiana in 2021, we had to pay full asking price and forgo an inspection as a nation of privileged teleworkers looking to upgrade their inner space drove the housing market into a frenzy. Many Americans lost a huge chunk of their gains in retirement funds when the pandemic clobbered the Dow. I fared worse, losing principal, because I'd had to forgo those gains. You see, back in 2016, the administration told me

I had to sell off all my retirement investments that were in the stock market as it was important I not be seen as potentially benefiting from any policy recommendations I made. Consequently, I missed out on the bear market that occurred from 2016 to 2020, which padded many people's accounts prior to the devastating losses that resulted from the pandemic.

Anyone who has lost their health insurance after losing a job knows how stressful that can be. The situation is even worse if they or anyone in their family has underlying medical conditions, like my wife and I both do. My job search took far longer than expected, as many potential employers feared reprisals for even talking to me, because I had been in the Trump administration. I literally went from being the Nation's Doctor to my entire family, including my wife with stage four cancer, being uninsured and unable to see a doctor. I could've gotten insurance via the government version of COBRA, but it's not as simple or affordable as people like to believe. Due to the cost and the hassle (you have to prepay for several months at a time, and that cost would be non-refundable even if I got a job during that timeframe), we made the same decision that many Americans do every day. We decided to roll the dice and go uninsured until we could again access employer-provided health insurance.

Fortunately, after eight months of searching, I found a good fit. I was asked by Purdue University to be their very first director of health equity initiatives. Some in the media have portrayed this job as a political gift from former Purdue president (and former Republican governor) Mitch Daniels. However, credit must go to the board of trustees to whom he reported for seeing *past* the politics and recognizing the value in having a former state health commissioner and a Black former US surgeon general to help advance their health equity work. Because of the politics, their move was seen as daring (and even by some as unjustified).

I paid a high price for my service in other ways too. Increased stress, lack of sleep, and a very demanding schedule caused my health to decline during the years I was US surgeon general. This was all the more significant when added to my already pre-existing conditions. I'm now on two blood pressure medications, a diabetes medication, and two asthma medications, among others. Hateful messages and death threats were sometimes left on my direct voicemail or even hand-delivered to my home mailbox, which didn't exactly help my stress level. I was called racial epithets regularly—most often, ironically, by the very people who proclaim to hate racism and bullying. Plus, I dealt with family disruption. My wife was too often left alone to do the parenting, take care of our home, and battle metastatic cancer, often going to doctor appointments and treatments alone, while I was working on behalf of our Nation. My kids had to leave friends, school, and the only home they knew—our family suffered greatly from the upheaval. They moved to DC only to face constant questions and criticisms about their dad and to, at times, be bullied themselves because of it.

I've had audiences discourage their institutions from asking me to come and speak and threaten to protest if I did. Many people feel I deserved this treatment (and have said as much, loudly, on social media and in print) because of their assumptions about my political affiliation and their ignorance about many of the issues highlighted in this book. But even if you feel *I* deserved death threats and hateful messages and the fear of getting sick or hurt while uninsured because of my public service, imagine how it made my wife feel. Imagine how my kids felt. Then ask yourself if you'd risk subjecting your family to such treatment for the sake of serving your country?

I list my complaints not because I seek pity but to make a crucial point. *If good people fear they will be attacked and their families will be hurt as a result of choosing to be public servants, we will only continue to severely drain the pool of highly competent and compassionate individuals in important policy positions.* We are already seeing a mass exodus of public health workers on the state and local levels. These positions are getting harder to fill and remaining open longer. Is this partisan and vitriolic environment—an environment we all contribute to—causing us to ask too much of potential public servants (and their families)?

Despite the hardships my family and I had to endure during my time as US surgeon general, I do not regret agreeing to serve my country as the Nation's Doctor. I'm often asked if I could go back in time, would I do it again? I believe deeply in our country and in the importance of service to her, so my answer is always an immediate and emphatic yes. That said, I hope all the suffering we went through as a country wasn't in vain. There are many lessons to be learned that can make us stronger, healthier, and more equitable in how we treat each other. Now more than ever, we must break through the BS and the bias to learn how we can best protect ourselves from COVID-19 and future health crises.

• CHAPTER 12 •

PROTECTING YOURSELF AND YOUR FAMILY

THROUGHOUT THIS BOOK, YOU'VE LEARNED the importance of layering protections to prevent harm from COVID-19. Sometimes, those layers are dictated by where you live and local policy decisions, but sometimes they are determined, in part, by personal choices. I've based my guidance here on the known science, showing you how I think about keeping myself and my loved ones safe—particularly in a pandemic. By following this advice, you too can navigate a confusing, political, and always-evolving onslaught of information.

IDENTIFY TRUSTED AND KNOWLEDGEABLE RESOURCES FROM WHOM YOU CAN GET YOUR HEALTH QUESTIONS ANSWERED

As SARS–CoV-2, the virus that causes COVID-19, continues to mutate, one of the most important things you can do is establish (or maintain) a steady relationship with a primary care provider. Doing so can help you optimize your baseline health, which is critical for fighting off new threats you may encounter. Just as importantly, it means you'll have a trusted source you can go to when you have questions about current and ever-changing health recommendations or recent pharmaceutical innovations.

Being adequately informed is your most important first line of defense.

Though the CDC has been criticized by the public and in this book, I still believe in (and follow) their guidance and that of my state and local health department on topics ranging from how to control my blood pressure to which vaccinations my kids and I should get. The CDC isn't perfect—it's run by humans, after all—but they are more reliable and accountable than your favorite podcaster, your Uncle Joe on Facebook, the meme you read, or the email you've just been forwarded.

PAY ATTENTION TO THE NUANCES IN PUBLIC HEALTH ADVISORIES ABOUT WHO IS MOST AT RISK

At some point, it falls on you to ascertain if you or someone you're caring for is at high risk for a bad outcome and to take appropriate action. You might be at risk because you're older, obese, immunocompromised, have a mental illness, or have comorbidities (for me, it's asthma and high blood pressure). Don't let misleading or outright false messages ones like "only old people die from COVID-19" cause you to ignore *your* unique risks. At the same time, be cautious about letting heightened fears about COVID-19 cause you to forgo precious time with friends and family or to avoid enjoyable, healthy activities. COVID-19 can absolutely kill you but so can isolation and lack of opportunities to support your physical and mental health.

Our immune systems degrade as we age, but there are robustly healthy seventy-year-olds with wonderfully strong immune systems and seven-year-olds whose immune systems have been weakened by preexisting medical conditions. We don't know why someone who is vaccinated and fully boosted, healthy, young, and fit can contract COVID-19 and be miserably sick for weeks while someone older, obese, and not up to date with their boosters contracts it and experiences only transient, mild symptoms. My wife's ninety-six-year-old grandfather contracted COVID-19 early in the pandemic and was out playing golf two weeks later. He's still alive today, and despite his prior infection, I'm happy to say he chose to get vaccinated because he's at higher risk. (And you should know that "hybrid" immunity—having been infected and vaccinated—has been found in multiple studies to be more protective than either infection or vaccination alone.)[138] But while weighing our individual risks, it's important not to ignore population-level statistics about which groups are getting sick and dying at higher rates. It's like Vegas: you may be on a hot streak now, but keep gambling and the house eventually wins. And you may be more—or less—at risk for acute hospitalization or death from COVID-19 or for long COVID-19 than you think. Far too many people don't realize they have an underlying condition that makes them more likely to experience a severe case of COVID-19—for example, undiagnosed depression. Talk with your doctor about your risks and how to reduce them.

BUILD AND MAINTAIN YOUR IMMUNITY BY PAYING ATTENTION TO PROPER DIET AND NUTRITION

Remember, obesity is an independent risk factor for poor outcomes if you contract COVID-19. Obesity, and consuming the types of food that predispose a person to it, also puts you at increased risk for diseases like diabetes, high blood pressure, and heart disease, which in turn puts you at higher risk for hospitalization and death from COVID-19, the flu, and whatever Mother Nature hits us with next. Try to consume more healthy foods, like fruits and vegetables, and enjoy less healthy foods in moderation. (Full disclosure: I love a good burger and fries, but I try to make such foods a treat versus a habit.)

Further, try to maintain balance in your diet to avoid nutritional deficiencies that can put you at risk for COVID-19 and other diseases. Maintaining adequate vitamin D levels year-round, especially when you have darker skin (and when you live in northern US states that experience less sunlight), is essential. I wish the task force had had the bandwidth to take up this topic more meaningfully. While scientific debate continues about the impacts of vitamin D supplementation on COVID-19 risk, we know vitamin D plays a crucial role in maintaining robust immunity. Many people of color lack sufficient levels and don't realize it, yet darker skin (and living far from the equator) makes it harder to absorb vitamin D from sunlight.[139] We also know that vitamin D deficiency is correlated with higher rates of cancer, heart disease, and more.

The bottom line is that adhering to a diet that limits calories and ensures nutritional balance can help you survive not just COVID-19 but an array of other diseases.

TRY TO LIMIT MISUSE OF HARMFUL SUBSTANCES

"Avoid or limit smoking, vaping, drinking, and drug use" is one of my mantras, and it should be no surprise, given the surgeon general has a warning label on many of these products. If you make a choice to engage in any of these activities, I encourage you to track your use because it may constitute a bigger part of your lifestyle than you think, especially when you're under stress (all these behaviors increased during the pandemic). Learn healthy ways to manage your stress. Having alternative, healthier ways to mitigate stress makes it easier to avoid unhealthy outlets like drinking or smoking/vaping tobacco or marijuana. Identify your own stressbusting tools (for me, it's exercise, meditation, and being outside) and look into new, healthy stress/anxiety/anger relievers you can add to your list. Limit the news you consume—particularly the political news—and choose news sources that are less likely to trigger a stress response (I admittedly need to better heed my own advice on that one). Avoiding stress, especially if that stress is coming from too much social media or television, is part of being your healthiest self.

MANAGE YOUR UNDERLYING CHRONIC CONDITIONS

High blood pressure is often called the silent killer because it's common not to feel its effects until it's too late. There were many silent killers during the pandemic, in the form of underlying and uncontrolled chronic diseases. These led to worse outcomes for those who were infected and even those who weren't. Again, more people died from uncontrolled blood pressure in 2020 than from COVID-19.[140] If your doctor has prescribed a treatment for a chronic disease like hypertension, adhere to your treatment plan. If you're having difficulty following your doctor's advice, talk to her or him, and try to work out a way to adjust (or afford) things so that you can more easily comply. The best medical advice in the world does you no good if you don't (or can't) follow the treatment plan.

CHECK YOUR BIASES

As we've discussed, to process new information and protect our health, it's vital that we recognize our biases, whether they are political or in favor of or against a particular policy or treatment recommendation. It's easy to experience confirmation bias— cherry picking facts that fit your opinion or viewpoint. Also, it's important to remember we all are both victims of, and contributors to, the monetization of conflict and division. People make money and build their brands when you like, share, and comment on social media posts that incite fear or anger or when you read or watch news that elicits such reactions, but the algorithms are only selling what we all are willingly buying. We face enough stress and confusion without adding to it by unnecessarily consuming and amplifying alarmist posting and reporting. When we the people recognize we are being played and change our own behaviors, the media and politicians will be forced to follow suit.

COMMUNICATE MORE RESPECTFULLY AND EFFECTIVELY ABOUT HEALTH, FOSTERING THE RELATIONSHIPS YOU'VE BUILT WITH OTHERS

When health conversations (or debates) arise among you and people you know, consider affirming others in expressing themselves on an important topic and take time to really listen before correcting them. Strive to learn more about the person's perspective, not just to prepare for a counterattack. There may be more thought and legitimate reasoning behind someone's position than you imagined, and you might be surprised to find you're not so far apart as you think. Better listening and more civil discourse can go a long way toward opening others' minds to new, better health information and to opening your own mind to perspectives and obstacles to health you've not considered. People need to know you care before they care what you know. (In July 2020, the *Washington Post* called me the nicest guy in Washington, but then openly questioned whether being nice was an effective approach in a pandemic.[141] Much as being combative can draw eyeballs to a screen, I still think we need more civil public—and private—discourse.)

PROTECT YOURSELF AND LOVED ONES FROM COVID BY REMEMBERING THE ACRONYMS PSA AND MTV

PSA is about assessing your *p*ersonal and *s*ituational risks so you can take appropriate *a*ction. MTV is about the tools you can use to protect yourself or your loved ones: *m*asking, *t*esting and *t*reatment, and *v*accines and *v*entilation.

P: Personal risk

When making health decisions such as whether to attend or skip an event based on the risk of getting infected with COVID-19 (or any other contagious disease or illness), ask yourself: Am I personally at high risk because of my comorbidities? What about the people with whom I live or work? Remember, you might not feel old at fifty or sixty, but that's when immunity starts to wane and comorbidities start to add up. If you work in a healthcare setting or live with someone who is vulnerable, you should consider your risk of contracting and passing on an infection to others, even if you don't personally see yourself as high risk. I make my decisions based not only on my own higher individual risk but also taking into account that my wife has cancer and I work with critically ill patients in the hospital. My personal risk assessment will not be the same as a healthy twenty-five-year-old who lives alone in an apartment and works from home.

S: Situational risk

Ask yourself: What's the situational risk I'm facing? What is the size of the crowd? Will I be inside or outside? Regardless, how's the ventilation? If outdoors, will we be closely packed together? If indoors, will windows and doors be open? Are the people I'm around likely to be up to date on their vaccinations, which protects us all to some degree (especially if they're recently boosted)? Will people be masking (and if so, will they be keeping their masks on or removing them to eat, drink, and converse?).

As an example, I feel somewhat safer at a medical conference than in other crowded indoor situations (like in an airport), because the people I'm around are more likely to be vaccinated and boosted. I feel safer removing my mask outdoors or in open ventilated areas, which is where I try to eat during conferences. I enjoy (and thus get mental health benefits from) going to sporting events with my kids and will attend a football or basketball game since they are typically either outside or in an arena with lots of open space. (I still wear a mask to and from my seat if community COVID-19 spread is elevated. The highest risk situations are when standing in admissions lines or waiting for concessions.) The bottom line is that risk varies by environment just as it does based on individual risk factors.

A: *Appropriate action*

Once you've done your own risk assessment, you can take appropriate action to protect yourself. Appropriate action might mean wearing a mask, deciding to take a rapid test, getting your booster shot (or encouraging a loved one to do so) before taking a vacation or attending a family gathering, or skipping an event altogether. As a society, we are blessed to have more tools than ever before to protect ourselves, but tools do nothing if they are never taken out of the toolbox.

Now let's look at MTV, which is how I think about the tools we can employ if we do decide to attend an event or engage in a higher-risk activity, depending on our individual and situational assessment.

M: *Masking*

Despite all the back and forth about this topic, masking, especially when using high-filtration masks like an N95 or KN95, remains one of the lowest cost and widely accessible tools we have for protecting ourselves against the spread of an array of viruses, including COVID-19. I use them often, especially when traveling. In fact, we now know that even before the availability of vaccines, hospital workers had lower rates of infection—despite caring for known COVID-19–positive patients—than the general public did, because they were wearing masks when they were at the highest situational risk. Much of the spread in hospitals occurred not in the rooms of COVID-19 patients but in nurses' and doctors' lounges, where the masks tended to come off. We must be honest about the fact that masks are far from perfect, especially if poorly constructed or fitted, but many studies have shown *any* mask you wear can provide some incremental benefit to you and/or others, especially if worn properly. The greater the number of people in a setting who wear masks, the more the benefit of masking increases. Additionally, masking can protect you not just from COVID-19 but other respiratory viruses like flu and RSV. That's why I wear a mask whenever I'm traveling through airports and on planes. I've not only been able to avoid COVID-19 when others around me have been infected, but I've also had far fewer seasonal infections than in the past.

T: Testing and treatment

Testing. Do you have timely access to testing if you become symptomatic or have a high-risk exposure? Do you keep rapid tests on hand? Rapid testing helps you know whether you should isolate and when to seek treatment. Some health departments still give out free at-home rapid tests, and if you have employer-provided health insurance, you may be able to (at least as of the writing of this book) get home tests for free. Talk to your local pharmacy or call your insurance company to find out.

Many pharmacies and health departments also offer free and convenient on-site COVID-19 testing. Armed with this knowledge, you should have a plan for testing if you're exposed to someone who informs you that they've tested positive for COVID-19. The time to think about where to get a test shouldn't be after you or a loved one are already sick. I maintain a supply of rapid antigen tests at my home and suggest that you do the same. I have used them often, including before attending group gatherings to ensure I'm not infected (but asymptomatic), which would cause others to be exposed. Recent FDA-approval of a combined COVID-19 and flu at home test means our ability to protect ourselves and loved ones may soon extend even beyond COVID-19.[142]

Treatments. COVID-19 treatments will (and must continue to) evolve, but right now, you should know that Paxlovid, an antiviral used to treat COVID-19 infections, lowers risk of hospitalization by over 90 percent.[143] However, it's crucial to remember that it needs to be taken soon (within 5 days) after infection. If you get sick or test positive, you'll want to have a plan for getting Paxlovid promptly, especially if you are at high risk. Too many people die every day from COVID-19 without knowing about or being able to access this lifesaving drug. Also know that you may have to self-advocate for you or a loved one to get treatment. The sad truth is that the medical system is failing us, and too many people are being denied antiviral treatment. I have had to intervene on behalf of more than one vulnerable family member to get them treated (unfortunately, most people don't have a former surgeon general they can call). Many pharmacies offer a test-to-treat program where you can test and, if found positive for COVID-19. have a telehealth session or on-site consultation with a medical provider to get Paxlovid—all without leaving the premises. The program is a potential pathway forward if you don't have a health provider or your health provider is reluctant to prescribe Paxlovid.

V: vaccines and ventilation

Vaccines. Vaccines are the absolute foundation of my own personal COVID-19 strategy, and being up to date on your vaccinations is far and away the most effective tool you have for protecting yourself from an infection that sends you to the hospital, turns into long COVID-19, or takes your life. No medical treatment is 100 percent safe, but the tradeoffs are clear. For the vast majority of people, getting available COVID-19 vaccines and boosters is safer and more reliable than getting repeatedly infected by COVID-19 (especially without the protection of vaccines). Improving baseline health helps, but getting up to date on vaccines and boosters remains the most quickly modifiable risk factor impacting your COVID-19 morbidity and mortality. As of this book's writing, the vast majority of those dying from COVID-19 have *not* been up to date on their vaccinations.

Also, vaccines are still somewhat effective (though not perfect) at preventing infection, especially within three to four months after injection. That might not seem like a long time, but currently available COVID-19 vaccines are as durable as the flu shot typically is in any given season (which is why it makes sense moving forward to time boosters with flu shots/likely seasonal spikes). The vaccines were amazingly good at preventing infections when they first were available, and they remain incredibly effective at preventing hospitalization and death, especially if boosted. While they might look as though they a failing in contrast to their initial performance, vaccines are still an incredibly powerful weapon against COVID-19.

Make sure you're also up-to-date with your annual flu shot and other recommended vaccines. As we saw in late 2022, even when COVID-19 doesn't take us down or overwhelm healthcare systems by itself, "syndemics" (simultaneous epidemics of more than one disease) of COVID-19 along with other viruses like flu,

RSV, and measles, can ruin a holiday or strain hospital capacity. So, prevent illness when you can by taking recommended vaccines. It's what I do for myself and my entire family.

If you or someone you love can't get vaccinated for medical reasons, it's all the more important that those around you are vaccinated to provide a protective "cocoon." We in the health field recommend this for anyone around newborn babies, for instance, as infants are too young to be vaccinated. Using other tools to protect against COVID-19 also becomes even more critical when you're around (or you are) someone who can't safely be vaccinated.

Ventilation. Ventilation remains the most underappreciated and underutilized tool for protecting ourselves against COVID-19. It should always be a consideration, both from a societal and a personal standpoint. I'd like to see more effort and investment in public (and private) buildings improving ventilation systems. Upgrades will protect people not just from COVID-19, but other infectious diseases like RSV and flu, as well as non-infectious health issues like allergies and asthma. Even as an individual, you have some power to protect yourself from COVID-19 by paying attention to ventilation. For example, you can decide not to eat inside a crowded restaurant and instead choose a place where you can eat outdoors. You can choose where and when to forgo a mask based on the openness and ventilation of the room you're in. You can even create your own personal home or work ventilation system. The Corsi–Rosenthal Box is a cleaning system you can fashion yourself using a box fan, MERV-13 furnace filters, and duct tape—materials you can find in your local hardware store for far less than it would cost to buy a fancy

HEPA filter machine. Improving your home ventilation can significantly reduce your exposure to indoor air particles, including ones that contain the coronavirus that causes COVID-19.[144] This can be extremely valuable when having guests over or when someone in your house does get COVID-19 and you are trying to keep it from spreading. Ventilation is an easy way to protect ourselves in a world in which we find ourselves exposed not just to COVID-19 but to an increasing array of airborne pollutants and infectious agents.

These personal tips and tools are how my family and I have survived COVID-19. None of them alone are effective all of the time, and most in my family have tested positive for COVID-19 at least once. But by taking precautions, we've been able to live reasonably normal lives while limiting repeat infections or family outbreaks. None of these strategies and suggestions are tools everyone can (or wants to) use in every situation. But as I've said repeatedly, when considering an activity you have to weigh risk and benefit—a constantly changing calculation—and layer the right tools to lower risk when possible. We all make different choices at different times based on our priorities as well as an array of external variables about risk, reward, and how we might insulate ourselves from harm.

Whatever choices you're considering, let's try to recognize, the misinformation, disinformation, politics, and hyperbole and leave it in the past. Let's use the lessons we've learned from a horrible pandemic that has claimed far too many lives, livelihoods, and relationships. That way, we can all better prepare ourselves for what lies ahead.

• CHAPTER 13 •

A SURGEON GENERAL'S WARNING

IN JANUARY 2022, UTAH JAZZ center Rudy Gobert tested positive for COVID-19. He quietly missed one game and endured five days of isolation from the team before returning to the court (akin to what would happen if he'd twisted an ankle). The media barely covered the story—a very different situation than when he had tested positive two years earlier, on March 11, 2020. Then, Gobert was abruptly pulled from the court on live television. The ripple effects included the entire NBA shutting down and then the NCAA's "March Madness," one of the most watched and most lucrative events in sports, being canceled.

The contrast between what happened when he tested positive in 2020 and then again in 2022 shows how mightily the world had changed in just two years. This time, Gobert, like millions of Americans, was vaccinated.[145] This time, he had access to a reliable treatment: Paxlovid, which shortens the time one has symptoms and is infectious and lowers the risk of hospitalization and death by over 90 percent. This time, Gobert had rapid tests that he could take at home daily to determine promptly and definitively when he could safely reintegrate into work and society. Also, he could safely stay in his spacious home, with a private bathroom, while having access to all the food and resources he needed to isolate.

This story illustrates tremendous success and progress in our fight against COVID-19, yet it also highlights our tremendous and continued failure as a society. Unlike sports stars, millions of people can't access rapid testing or obtain Paxlovid. Too many Americans are not up to date on their vaccinations. Far too few can afford to lose five days or more to isolation because they can't do their jobs remotely or don't have sick leave. Many Americans' homes don't allow them to safely and comfortably isolate. And we're still inundated with COVID-related misinformation and disinformation—including the fallacy that a COVID-19 infection is guaranteed to be harmless and a mere mild inconvenience. In fact, Rudy Gobert, an elite athlete previously in peak health, experienced symptoms of long COVID-19 after his 2020 infection.[146] And while Gobert isolated in January 2022, the Delta and Omicron variants of COVID-19 surged so much that pediatric hospitalizations and deaths were at their highest level ever. One third of those children were healthy before catching COVID-19,[147] and most who were hospitalized were unvaccinated.[148]

If we don't learn our lessons, we are doomed to continue seeing high levels of avoidable sickness, hospitalizations, and deaths—as well as long COVID—and to repeat the same mistakes we've made throughout the pandemic. This impacts not just individuals but also our workforce and the economy at large. Several studies now show long COVID-19 is keeping significant numbers of US citizens from resuming their jobs.[149] We saw mistakes made again and again with repeat surges of COVID-19 and in 2022 with the mpox outbreak.

Throughout this book, I've mentioned some of my take-aways from experiences before, during, and after I served as US surgeon general. Some are big, and some are small. Some are for the individual, yet many are my ideas about changing systems and infrastructure. But the ten lessons I share in this chapter are relevant to everyone. Community leaders, school administrators, business managers, influencers, and everyday people are all in this together. Countless books and reports on COVID-19 delve deeply into some of these issues, but many of them haven't been highlighted enough, continue to be ignored, or don't deal with the root of the problem. You can't address an issue until you truly understand what caused it; you have to learn why a challenge keeps appearing over and over again. My hope is that you will look at things differently in the context of the stories in this book. My plea to you is to take them to heart, for all our sakes. Let's do better together so that we can all thrive.

LESSON 1: WE MUST TAKE PARTISANSHIP OUT OF PUBLIC HEALTH

When health officials and organizations come across as politically partisan, they immediately lose half their audience for important health messages. Belonging to groups of physicians dedicated to supporting a particular presidential candidate or being identified as "Trump's" or "Biden's" or any other president's surgeon general, CDC director, or special advisor is problematic for a public health advocate whose job is to engage everyone. Both Democrats and Republicans politicized COVID-19, and the Trump administration's response to it. For example, in 2020, Democrats far outspent Republicans in COVID-related political ads ($476 million to $159 million).[150] "Only we can fix COVID" was a centerpiece of 2020 Democratic campaigns. Yet even with full Democratic control of the White House, Congress, and federal public health machinery and the availability of a vaccine (as well as far more tests and PPE), many more died from COVID-19 in 2021 than in 2020 under the prior administration.[151] In a *New York Times* opinion piece called "9 Pandemic Narratives We're Getting Wrong," David Wallace-Wells wrote that, "The most consequential year of the pandemic in the United States was probably not 2020 but 2021," adding, "In the first year of the pandemic, the United States performed somewhat worse than some of its peers in the wealthy West but not that much worse[152]. We failed to stop the virus at the border, but so did most other countries in the world, and by the end of 2020, [America's] Covid-19 per capita death toll was near the European Union average…. But it was in the pandemic's second year[153] that the country really faltered."[154]

Now, this doesn't mean we should blame all 2021 COVID-19 deaths on "Democratic" policies any more than we should blame the 2020 ones on Republicans. But it does mean the real issues go far deeper than whether you were "Ridin' with Biden" or seeking to "Make America Great Again" on election day.

I saw up close how easy it is to compromise outreach to underserved communities when partisanship gets in the way. At one point, the White House partnered Dr. Fauci and me with celebrity spokespeople (like actor Dennis Quaid) to do interviews in which we discussed ways people could protect themselves and their communities from COVID-19. We knew celebrities could be quite influential with certain audiences, and I felt it was a great idea. I was overjoyed to sit down with African American gospel legend CeCe Winans. We were both hopeful we could get the word out to Black communities about how to safely worship and support others in your church community during the pandemic. This is exactly the kind of thing people you'd expect a surgeon general to do (and which the public complained the Trump administration wasn't doing enough of, in terms of outreach), no? Unfortunately, Ms. Winans got ripped by the Black community for supposedly promoting Donald Trump and his administration (though we never once mentioned Trump or politics in our conversation), and she was falsely accused of being paid for the interviews.[155] The same happened with Dennis Quaid, who said of his conversation with Dr. Fauci, "No good deed goes unpoliticized."[156] It makes no sense to claim you want people, especially those who disagree with you politically, to spread the facts about COVID-19 and then attack the very people who are trying to help educate the public. At least not if your true motive is helping support healthy communities.

Of course, blaming media and social media personalities for their flaws when we're the ones who consume and share their negative news stories isn't fair. We all have a responsibility to recognize and take the partisanship out of public health. We must stop pointing fingers and demonizing people's choices, especially when it comes more from a place of partisanship than scientific grounding. Let's be better listeners as well as communicators. And I hope I've convinced you to consider and respect the challenges of health officials who are put in difficult positions because of politics and yet stick it out for the sake of serving their communities.

Politics and health policy have become so intertwined and so divisive that now they even permeate our schools and workplaces. People scream and threaten each other at school board meetings about which health measures we should take to protect our kids. Casual workplace conversations in the breakroom suddenly go silent when someone known to have different beliefs about pandemic mitigation walks by. My advice is that if you're a business leader or school board member hoping to avoid the politicization and vilification of health policies, consider having early, open, and frequent conversations to discuss the what and the why of such recommendations—putting the reasoning before the policy, and not the other way around. And whenever possible, try to allow for flexibility and choices when setting policies. That way, you increase the likelihood of cooperation rather than rebellion. Everyone wants kids to learn, businesses to thrive, workers to find jobs, and an end to divisiveness. Start with that common ground and focus on listening, collaborating, and coming up with solutions to problems instead of tearing each other down and trying to "defeat" the other side.

Finally, the interplay of politics and health isn't just local or even national. It's also global, as we saw with China sharing the genetic sequence of the virus but not infection data (and not cooperating fully with investigations into COVID's origins). We need more international cooperation regarding health information and resources. We are all in this together, every human being. And there's a version of the golden rule embedded in just about every spiritual tradition around the globe. Let's do what we can to help those less fortunate, whether we promote vaccine access in poorer nations or avoid hoarding supplies when there's a crisis.

LESSON 2: SCIENCE AND HEALTH LITERACY MUST IMPROVE

One of the fallouts of the COVID-19 pandemic was an increased resistance to following the advice of recognized health experts. For many, "do your own research" has become a mantra. While I fully support people educating themselves on health and risk, too many aren't equipped with the tools to understand what responsible, reliable research involves. Of course, experts aren't perfect. But unlike people whose main expertise lies in their ability to build a following for their YouTube and TikTok channels, health experts are not only more learned in the basic science, but also trained to be at least somewhat more aware of and to address their biases. They are less likely to embrace and play into them (and profit from them) like many in the media and on social media do. Also, most people trained in our current scientific best practices strongly believe in the importance of peer review and consensus and are subject to at least some degree of fact checking and accountability.

I'm not saying we should never question "experts"—far from it. The nature of science is that our knowledge and understanding of the world are always evolving, so we must always question and test previous beliefs. However, the pandemic increased the breadth and pace of the emergence of new knowledge, meaning it is even more vital for us to apply appropriate scientific standards to our assessment of new findings and we trust the process—even as we question beliefs.

The pandemic exposed our lack of math and science literacy in the US as far too high. Internationally, the US ranks nineteenth in science and thirtieth in math.[157] Many people don't understand basic statistics yet feel fully capable of understanding complex research studies, which rely on statistical analysis for validity. Just look at the number of people on Facebook or Twitter on any given day quoting a study and insisting it unquestionably supports their beliefs or preferred policies. Often, they fail to understand who was included in the study and who funded it, and they don't notice or care that the study included only sixteen people or that it includes specific disclaimers about how it actually does *not* support a particular conclusion. Half of adults read below the sixth-grade level, [158] yet many of those same adults will insist that they (or their favorite podcaster) know more about a topic than a doctor or scientist who has spent their life studying it, because they "have done their research."

As new scientific data comes in, our understanding of health challenges and best treatments will change, which means guidelines must change in response. The collective outcry against COVID-19 guidelines being updated would not have been as intense if more Americans understood the scientific process and been better at recognizing misinformation and disinformation. It also wouldn't have been as intense if the scientific community was more skilled at communicating with the public simply, apolitically, and with a healthy dose of humility.

Misinformation and disinformation about the effectiveness of hydroxychloroquine and ivermectin as treatments for COVID-19 was hard to combat. People often don't understand how clinical trials, research studies, and journals work and that the plural of "anecdotes" isn't "evidence," and that "this happened to my cousin's boyfriend's mom" doesn't equate to population-level certainty.

A lack of understanding about clinical trials also led many to think vaccine development was rushed and important steps were skipped, which as I've said, was far from the case—in fact, the COVID-19 vaccines are far and away *the* most scrutinized medical products in history. Clinical trials have several stages during which medications are tested to determine effectiveness and appropriate dosages, and the COVID-19 vaccines were no exception.

When doctors didn't know how to treat COVID-19 or were short on options for the sick and dying, they tried some medications that were already available, prescribing them "off-label." That practice is common, especially when there is an immediate need to treat someone. Initial reports about hydroxychloroquine were promising, but the promise didn't stand up to scientific scrutiny so we don't recommend this medication as a tool to combat COVID-19. An interesting example in the other direction is using steroids to treat hospitalized COVID-19 patients. Previously, doctors thought giving steroids to someone with a severe flu-like respiratory infection was bad medicine. However, a few anecdotes and off-label efforts led to larger studies, and prescribing steroids *is* now a best practice for in-hospital COVID-19 treatment. That's the way the process is supposed to work, to optimize both efficacy and safety.

Also, people may not realize that sound research studies are typically subject to consensus. Anyone can post their "research" study on a website. To be accepted by a high-quality medical journal, a study has to undergo rigorous peer review to lessen the likelihood that it isn't flawed (by innocent mistake or, as in the case of discredited anti-vaxxer Andrew Wakefield, with his full knowledge of its problems, which he didn't disclose).[159] If reviewers discover problems with the study, the authors can make changes to improve or clarify it and resubmit it. Additionally, the authors must disclose who funded the study in case there might be a conflict of interest or financial incentives that could cause the researchers to be biased, which might lead them to distort the study's findings. Too many "studies" are touted today, and sadly used to guide policy, without being subject to this same level of review and scrutiny.

Because there is so much new information every day to digest, doctors rely on quality clinical trials published in peer-reviewed journals to guide treatment recommendations and decisions. If you're intrigued by the results of a study showing that patients' health improved after they received a particular treatment, you should feel more assured if it appeared in a respected medical journal. Feel less assured if you only find it on a website. And always—*always*—discuss any new medications you are considering with your doctor or trusted health provider.

When looking at studies, pay attention to who the participants were. For example, notice whether their demographics (age, sex, race, other medical issues, etc.) match yours. This latter point was also an issue throughout the pandemic: Even a well-conducted study may only apply to specific groups, especially if the study was small. After Operation Warp Speed began, Dr. Fauci, NIH director Francis Collins, and I recognized that lack of diversity in early trials of COVID-19 vaccines was an issue, so I became involved in broadening the pool of participants.[160] If we want to achieve healthcare equity, diversity in clinical trials is critical. It helps us improve the integrity of our scientific process.

Many pride themselves on citing statistics and facts to support their positions, but are they cherry-picking and being taken in by misinformation (if not disinformation) to avoid changing a narrative that appeals to them? Some people, often believing that everyone in public health or working in a pharmaceutical company only cares about money and power and not about other people, reject information from respected (and vetted) sources, especially when that information doesn't confirm their biases. Be skeptical of claims made by outliers, even if those outliers are physicians. It doesn't mean they are wrong, but it does mean their claims should be subject to further scrutiny before amplifying or extrapolating from them.

As for knowing which experts to trust, we should acknowledge our natural tendency to cast people into the roles of persecutor, rescuer, and victim. As I said before, doing that leads to distorted narratives. If the medical community is the enemy and people who don't "do their own research" are the victims, there's a temptation to see yourself as a rescuer, above making mistakes or exhibiting bias. You might think you're sharing reliable information with others when you're not. It's tempting to project this same rescuer narrative onto an outlier physician. Confirmation bias (seeing what you expect to see), normalcy bias (which leads people to disbelieve or minimize threat warnings), and other forms of cognitive bias affect us all. Biases make the brain work more efficiently, but they can cause us to overlook important facts and context. We need to reflect on our perceptions to see where we might need to be more open-minded and flexible in our thinking.

Finally, we must help our kids catch up in scientific literacy. We were already behind much of the developed world pre-pandemic, and our children have only fallen further behind because of how the pandemic affected their schooling (more on that shortly). Again, as Surgeon General Jocelyn Elders says, "it's hard to be healthy if you're not educated."

LESSON 3: WE HAVE TO ADDRESS THE PROBLEM OF MISINFORMATION AND DISINFORMATION

Misinformation and disinformation can cause people to reject protective and treatment measures (which we see with vaccine hesitancy and the low uptake of boosters and Paxlovid). They also are contributing to a deep mistrust of government, scientists, and public health officials—and can thus can actually lead to severe illness and death. In the US, life expectancy has dropped because of COVID-19, particularly so for African Americans and Native Americans.[161] While most people who are under age sixty and have no underlying risk factors experience only mild illness from COVID-19, remember, not everyone who has an underlying condition (such as high blood pressure or obesity) is aware of it. In fact, most American adults have at least one comorbid condition that puts them in a "high risk" category for COVID-19 complications. Further, we can't always predict who will have a severe case of COVID-19. And even if you initially develop only a moderate level of illness from COVID-19, you have a 20 percent chance of developing long COVID-19 (symptoms of COVID-19 that can linger for months or longer).[162] The

CDC estimates it will cost $9,000 a year to treat each case of long COVID-19, costing the US economy $528 billion annually.[163] In other words, misinformation and disinformation cost us dearly—not just in morbidity and mortality, but also in dollars and cents.

Unfortunately, we sometimes push people towards the misinformers. It's frustrating to have low COVID-19 vaccination and boost rates. Yet as I said, public health officials, political leaders, community leaders, and friends and relatives of the unvaccinated need to recognize that many so-called anti-vaxxers are, more accurately, just vaccine-*hesitant*. If that describes you, talk with a trusted doctor or nurse practitioner about your risks. Misinformation and disinformation can, and often do, fill the void when those conversations are absent, or when people are shamed for vaccine hesitancy.

We also must acknowledge that some in the scientific community spread misinformation, even if they didn't mean to. Public health officials and those of us in the medical community have to be honest about what the science does and doesn't tell us, even when the information we give might irritate and anger people or could cause them to take actions we might want to discourage. We also need to be careful not to gaslight people whose personal, lived experience contradicts what we know—or believe we know—about diseases, treatments, and side effects of medical treatments and vaccines. People need to feel that they're being heard by the public health community and not shamed for their situations and choices. We can better address concerns when we truly listen and empathize, building instead of eroding trust in health authorities. One way to do that is to be sure they know about the vaccine adverse effects reporting system (VAERS) so that they can report health problems they suspect could be side effects of vaccines.

Another key to fighting misinformation and disinformation is for public health officials to partner with influencers to spread accurate health information. For instance, we could have made better use of America's obsession with sports and partnered with athletes to counteract misinformation and disinformation being shared on social media. I've always said LeBron James, Patrick Mahomes, or Aaron Judge can be more effective at changing health behaviors than the US surgeon general. That said, such outreach can backfire if a partisan narrative gets imposed on the efforts.

LESSON 4: WE NEED BETTER DATA, MORE QUICKLY

As I said in a March 2022 *USA Today* op-ed, I remember when at the White House in 2020, it seemed the US healthcare system was close to collapse. How many people were actually in the hospital with COVID-19? How many ICU beds did we have available? How many ventilators? "We don't really know," was the answer from top health officials. "Why the (bleep) not?" bellowed President Trump. We didn't have the infrastructure to facilitate or the authority to compel hospitals and healthcare institutions to report that information to the government—so most didn't. As I often say to audiences, we were driving down a dark road at night with both headlights out, turning the steering wheel only after we hit something.[164]

At the beginning of the pandemic, the CDC couldn't access data like COVID-19 test results and hospital capacity assessments. A national public health emergency declaration played a significant role in temporarily easing these issues. The declaration gave the HHS the authority to require reporting of the testing and hospitalization data that local, state, and federal public health officials use to guide our collective pandemic response. As various aspects of the emergency declaration have been lifted, those federal authorities and the data flows they enable have also disappeared.

The pandemic has revealed many faults in our public health response capabilities. The CDC now has no direct legal authority to lead and coordinate what or how much of our national public health data is collected. The result is a fragmented system with inconsistent reporting across fifty states and thousands of jurisdictions. Moreover, to access that data, the CDC must negotiate data-use agreements with each jurisdiction and for each public health matter.[165]

Our national public health operating picture is inefficient and can't support the modern, interoperable data-sharing environment that we need. Collecting and analyzing data is the very foundation of our national ability to prepare for and respond to future and ongoing public health threats.

Unifying the nation around a common approach to collecting and sharing data will benefit the entire public health ecosystem. We should support a data infrastructure which public health partners at the local, state, and national levels can access, and it must be timely, representative, and adhere to privacy standards. Now is not the time to go backward on an issue as important as our ability to see, collect, and share critical public health data. Health officials, governors, and the president of the United States should never again have to ask why the (bleep) we don't know what's going on when we're in a health emergency.

We also must improve the breadth of data coming into those surveillance systems, using modalities such as sewage surveillance, and we need real-time dashboards so we can see the road ahead rather than just reacting to the bump we have already hit.

LESSON 5: WE NEED TO RETHINK AND RESTRUCTURE OUR FEDERAL PUBLIC HEALTH EMERGENCY RESPONSE SYSTEM

To her credit, former CDC director, Rochelle Walensky, acknowledged the CDC didn't perform adequately during the pandemic under either administration. In her words, the CDC has been "responsible for some pretty dramatic and pretty public mistakes, from testing to data to communications."[166] Regardless of how the CDC might be restructured, and regardless of whether or not a new government agency is created or more authority is shifted to other agencies, we need to foster a culture of swift action in a crisis. Waiting weeks and months for data analysis, recommendations, and responses related to a rapidly spreading infectious disease is completely unacceptable.

In my opinion, we need to increase involvement of ASPR and work to better delineate the when, what, and how of an emergency response hand off. Pandemics are never declared with the first ten or even ten thousand cases. Every year, we have multiple new viruses or mutations that arise somewhere. The CDC watches and studies local outbreaks, and most are eventually contained or fizzle out. The challenge is that there is no clear point at which someone says, "We need to shift from a surveillance and regional response mindset" (a mindset typical for the

CDC) "and adopt a widespread crisis/pandemic response type of mindset" (a way of operating that the CDC struggles with). But what I'm describing is exactly what ASPR's mission is. Some in the media have complained that the CDC was "sidelined" in the Trump administration. Again, our national response to COVID-19 became much more functional when the CDC took on more of a support versus front line response role, and when ASPR and FEMA—agencies designed for and accustomed to the pace and, at times, the uncertainty of an emergency response—became more involved. At any other time, ASPR's Bob Kadlec, who helped coordinate the safe evacuation and redistribution across the country of thousands aboard the *Diamond Princess*, would've been given the Presidential Medal of Honor for his efforts. That situation could have been an absolute disaster of a national superspreader event with catastrophic consequences, especially at a stage when we had no vaccines or treatments. ASPR has better relationships with hospital and healthcare emergency response partners on the state and local level than the CDC does. They even work more closely with the crisis response leaders in state and local health departments.

Let's also better monitor the stockpile and the stock rotation so that supplies like masks, gowns, and gloves aren't rodent-infested or past their expiration dates. Let's review whether current storage facilities are in the best locations should we experience another fifty-state outbreak. Let's look to a reallocation model in a crisis instead of just relying on the "stockpile" model. There's no reason our national crisis distribution center system can't be as efficient as that of Amazon, which at many points throughout the pandemic could deliver an N95 mask to your front door—

whether it was your home or your local hospital—faster than the government could.

I'd like a commitment from Congress to incentivize having more PPE manufactured here in the US. Our response system was far too reliant on Chinese manufacturers and supply chains outside the US. The good news is that many in the US stepped up during the pandemic and proved we could manufacture masks, shields, hand sanitizer, and more right here in America. The bad news is that as soon as the pandemic supply crunch ended, healthcare systems returned to purchasing from the supplier offering the lowest cost versus the most-local supply. There are already many books and reports written on the specific policy changes that can and should occur to better prepare us for the next pandemic, but again, the overall lesson is that we can't keep relying on the same old dysfunctional infrastructure and response systems and expect that we will get different results. That has proven true no matter which administration is in charge during a pandemic.

LESSON 6: PUBLIC HEALTH OFFICIALS SHOULD NOT UNDERESTIMATE THE VALUE OF RELATIONSHIPS WHEN DEALING WITH HEALTH CRISES

Throughout my public health career, I've found building relationships is crucial when trying to solve problems. I experienced this when I was the Indiana State Health commissioner during the worst HIV-outbreak related to injection drug use in the history of the US. I could have managed things from our command center in Indianapolis. That would've been easier for me, my staff, and my family. Instead, I frequently traveled two hours each way to rural Scott County, Indiana, to personally experience their public health crisis up close. I did a ride-along with the local police chief. I learned how commonplace drug deals and prostitution were on the local streets. I met with church leaders and their parishioners, local doctors, pharmacists, and business owners. Over dinners and in rooms filled with metal folding chairs and tearful parents who had lost their children, I listened, and I let people know I understood why they were worried that a needle exchange might encourage drug use and enable people with substance use disorder. "My brother," I would start, "has substance use disorder and is incarcerated." That got their attention and allowed me to show them I truly heard and empathized with their concerns. Acknowledging common ground before beginning a difficult conversation rather than shaming and blaming has always been a helpful tool for me. Unfortunately, it's a tool we used far little during the pandemic.

Respect and earnest engagement is what got the people of Scott County from full-on reluctance to a place where they could consider a needle exchange. When they decided it was the right choice for them, *they* told the governor and explained how they came to this conclusion. In response, he agreed to use his executive authority to allow a syringe exchange (such programs were illegal in the state at the time). He then supported legislation to make such programs legal in the state. The Scott County model, in which people with injected drugs would be given clean syringes but also many other services, including referrals to treatment and recovery centers, led to successes that inspired other states. Many states not known for progressive politics, and that were largely against these types of harm reduction programs, adopted or adapted our model. It was an outcome I didn't expect—a ripple effect that helped countless people and prevented many more deaths. And it couldn't have happened without first building trust and relationships between the big-city health officials proposing the policies and the people on the ground who actually had to implement and live with them.

Now compare and contrast this experience to our pandemic response. In too many cases, the COVID-19 task force from their comfy perch in DC or the CDC scientists from their labs in Atlanta were making rules that people in communities far across America had to implement and live with, even when the consequences were very problematic. In many cases, the on-the-ground resources necessary to enact the theoretical or textbook guidelines weren't available. In other cases, the tradeoffs weren't fully and openly acknowledged and discussed. Shutting down schools limits potential viral spread in that environment, but what about the harms of missing out on educational opportunities and the socialization schools offer? According to an international survey of teachers conducted in 2021, "Teachers reported that students were an average of two months behind at the time of the survey, with low-income and at-risk students suffering higher setbacks...."[167] A report by UNESCO, UNICEF, and the World Bank shared similar findings and noted, "Reopening schools should be countries' highest priority. The cost of keeping schools closed is steep and threatens to hamper a generation of children and youth while widening pre-pandemic disparities."[168]

Consider the problem of other tradeoffs that were too often overlooked. Masking works, but what if someone is hard of hearing and relies on reading lips to navigate the world? Or what

if you "choose" to go to a large and fancy indoor gathering—
say, a White House Correspondents Dinner—and then you get
COVID-19? It's no problem now. You can just take Paxlovid,
right? Unfortunately, far too many people can't find a doctor who
will prescribe, a pharmacy that will dispense, or now, an insurer
that will cover it. It's no wonder the public became so angry with
federal health policymakers. They often seemed oblivious to the
reality most people faced when making everyday decisions.

When Dr. Birx, others on the COVID-19 task force, and I
visited communities in 2020, we saw the on-the-ground reality
and tried to have open and honest discussions in town hall settings. As a result, we developed better and more practical policies
and saw increased local understanding and adoption of those policies. Largely due to partisan politics, we are seeing fewer of these
types of visits from federal health leaders. Throughout most of
2021, they didn't visit states and didn't even meet with each other
face to face. (Many federal health officials worked remotely and
met virtually throughout 2021 and beyond, even as the White
House repeatedly said the situation had drastically improved
and the pandemic was "over.") And while Dr. Birx and I visited
most every state, red or blue, we rarely saw federal health officials talking about COVID-19 alongside Republican governors
when the administrations changed. Without those relationships,
preparing for and responding to the next pandemic will be very
challenging.

LESSON 7: WE NEED BETTER MESSAGING AND THE INFRASTRUCTURE AND RESOURCES TO SUPPORT IT

In 2022, the New York subway system featured posters approved by the health department that said when it came to masking, "You do you," and showed faces wearing masks on their chins and under their noses. This misguided endeavor to connect with the public was ripped by many, including yours truly. One such attempt at outreach that I regret and wish I could get a do-over on was in February of 2020. In the spirit of "health valentines" that public health advocates on social media were posting at the time, I tweeted, "Roses are red, violets are blue, risk is low for coronavirus but high for the flu." Unlike "You do you," this was widely considered to be an accurate statement by the public health community when I wrote it (we were in a terrible flu surge at that point, yet had almost no reported cases of COVID-19 in the US) and was consistent with WHO, CDC, and other major health organizations were saying. However, I must own the fact that it certainly didn't age well. People still question and attack my credibility based on that tweet—a tweet someone experienced in public communication might have warned me against posting. The lesson is twofold. First, being a high-level official or agency comes with great scrutiny and responsibility, so choose your words wisely and think about how they might sound not just today but in the future. Second, how you say it is just as important as what you say. In trying to be humorous or engaging, you can't sacrifice accuracy and clarity.

I think the US surgeon general, the CDC director, and other highly visible members of the HHS should have professional communications experts on staff who can help craft messages, and these experts should be a step removed from the White House. My own challenges getting help with messaging reminds me that too often, we didn't have the right people for the right tasks. Too frequently, we had scientists crafting public messages, doctors who didn't understand public health who were creating population level policy, and policymakers and politicians sticking their nose in the science.

Also, I understand the desire to keep hopes high and not instill panic, but it's a bad idea for politicians to create imaginary goalposts and then move them (such as suggesting that a virus might be gone by Easter, which President Trump did). It erodes trust in the administration and, more importantly, in public health officials. People need clarity—and honesty—about what's happening.

We also need to have more of a regional communications approach during a national health crisis. Just as tornadoes or hurricanes don't hit everywhere at the same time (which is why we don't tell people in North Dakota to take shelter or evacuate when a hurricane is heading for Florida), neither does a virus. Messaging in March 2020 about hospitals being overrun was appropriate for the Northeast but fell flat (and led to distrust) in Norman, Oklahoma. And we need to have a better communications plan for checkpoints and exits—what happens after "fifteen days to slow the spread?" When should a pandemic be declared "over," and what does that mean for Americans? In both medicine and public health, we know that people eventually check out if their treatment plan comes across as too demanding and never-ending, especially if they can't see progress or too often wonder "What's the point?" However, we also know that most diseases don't just disappear. They require long-term and sometimes life-long, treatment. What should the public health message be about the "end" of a pandemic when thousands are being infected, and hundreds are still dying daily?

Also, and again, I now realize that it's not just the message that matters but the messenger (and the company that messenger keeps). Addressing Black and Brown communities while frequently appearing next to someone viewed by many as racist was always going to be problematic. We (and I) needed to work harder to separate the health messages from the politics and presence of the president. And the same holds true (yet in opposite directions) for the current administration and health officials. It's hard to be seen as neutral or apolitical while standing next to the world's most recognized political figure.

LESSON 8: WE CAN'T BE A HEALTHY NATION WITHOUT HEALTH EQUITY

While equality is an admirable goal, it is often an incomplete one. That's why we need to understand and embrace the concept of health *equity*—making sure people are getting the resources they need to make healthy choices. The pandemic shed light on inequitable access to vaccines, testing, treatments, and the internet, which was sorely needed for virtual schooling or telehealth appointments and remote work. Further, too many could not work from home or take off work if sick. As of the writing of this book, deaths from COVID-19 are still topping a thousand a week. The number has now become background noise in our rush to return to the old normal—unless you're in a group at high risk for COVID-19 hospitalization and death.

We see something similar when hurricanes hit the South. Those who can simply pack up and leave, do. Those who are victimized belong to the same groups as those most victimized by COVID-19—the ones who can't just leave (The most concentrated outbreaks throughout 2020 were in correctional facilities, nursing homes, and food processing plants). We see it in our diabetes, cancer, and heart disease statistics and in homelessness after a devastating storm or flood. And despite the opioid epidemic receiving more attention in recent years as it hit more of White and suburban America, we've seen broken homes and deadly overdoses for decades in Black and Brown communities. We must do better at acknowledging, studying, and addressing health inequities, or we will continue to see more of the same harm with future health crises, no matter who is in charge.

LESSON 9: WE HAVE TO REMEMBER THAT ECONOMICS AND HEALTH ARE INTERTWINED

The top layer of Abraham Maslow's pyramid of human needs is self-actualization—that is, being the best (and healthiest) you that you can be. The next layer down is "esteem," which includes respect by and for others. Neither of these is a priority until the needs of the lower layers of the hierarchy (food, shelter, safety, etc.) are met. For too many people, particularly that half of all Americans who don't have $400 saved for an emergency, thinking about those top two layers is a luxury they both figuratively and literally can ill afford. It takes money to house yourself and your family and put clothes on your backs and food on the table. That's one of the main (and least talked about) reasons health is not a priority for most Americans. Buying costly fruits and vegetables from Whole Foods, taking time off from work to see the doctor, or purchasing COVID-19 tests and N95 masks is impossible for far too many Americans—let alone worrying about doing what's best for strangers.

When the economy's bad, it's hard for people to think about anything but making ends meet. That's why we need to talk more about health as an economic issue and economics as a health issue. As a member of the COVID-19 task force, I advocated for rent protections and financial support from the government so that people could more easily stay home during the pandemic. I've argued for the need to provide free at-home tests and high-filtration masks for those who can't afford them. If we want people to do right by society, we've got to do right by them, by ensuring that looking out for someone's health isn't being pitted against meeting their basic needs and obligations. It's also why as surgeon general I put out a first-of-its-kind report, called Community Health and Economic Prosperity,[169] making the business (as opposed to the medical) case for healthy, educated, and safe, "high opportunity" communities. Healthy communities offer employers a larger and more productive workforce and lower healthcare expenses. In other words, more health leads to more wealth.

The premise of my unique surgeon general's report was that partnerships among communities, nonprofits, and businesses can lead to better health and increased prosperity. One example we detail in the report is Greyston Bakery in New York. Chef Bernie Glassman often hired people with little to no work experience, including those with records of drug use and incarceration. New employees serve an apprenticeship for six to nine months, at which point they can join a union. Sometimes, an employee starts by showing up late or missing work often. Instead of firing them, Greyston has an onsite social worker meet with them to determine if they need help with childcare, threat of eviction, domestic violence, or some other issue that can be addressed with the help of Greyston's partner, Westchester Community Services. Another business example is UnitedHealthcare (UHC), which partnered with community organization La Causa to acquire low-income rental housing units in Phoenix, Arizona, for UHC clients. Inpatient hospital costs have been slashed in half, and emergency room visits have been reduced, all signs of better health care.

We know that health influences the ability to work. As a society, we are obligated to give more people better opportunities to make good choices about their health. Recognizing the connection between health and wealth is both a personal and a societal imperative.

LESSON 10: LACK OF US HEALTH RESILIENCE COMPROMISES FUTURE CRISIS RESPONSES

That the US did far worse than comparable European countries in protecting ourselves from the spread of the virus, especially in 2020, is a myth.[170] Countries such as France and Germany have documented similar or greater infection rates. What differs is what happened *after* people got infected. The infection fatality rate—the chances that you'd die if you became infected—was twice as high in the US as in Germany and France.[171] This is unlikely to be due to the quality of health care delivered to the sick. The availability of healthcare, even considering the unconscionably high numbers of people who don't have health insurance or easy access to a doctor in the US, probably isn't the cause. We need to look at Italy—the one country where the healthcare system truly broke during the pandemic—to better understand why our infection fatality rate was so high.

During Italy's worst surge, people were dying of COVID-19 in hospital hallways and too often couldn't get into a hospital, yet Italy's infection fatality rate was still ultimately lower than that of the US. Why?

First, America is more obese and has a higher chronic disease burden than other wealthy (and numerous not-so-wealthy) nations, including Italy. We have higher rates of cancer, diabetes, high blood pressure, lung disease, substance abuse, and pretty much any disease or risk factor that puts one in danger of death from COVID-19. This reality can't be quickly addressed, and America has not shown it is willing to address it meaningfully. Doing so would mean taking on politically dicey issues like what kinds of food we subsidize and how much money we should invest in creating green spaces in blighted communities. The second reason America's infection fatality rate is higher than other nations', especially post-2020, is because we have been chronically under-vaccinated. While we as a nation are at 80 percent of people who have received two doses of an mRNA vaccine or one dose of the Johnson & Johnson vaccine, we achieved that mark far later than most European countries did, despite having far earlier access to vaccines. Subsequently, we've also had low uptake of boosters that help to maintain or increase protection in the face of new variants.

Vaccines are one of the planet's top lifesaving innovations, and a vaccinated society is a resilient one. The US military has long noted infection from vaccine-preventable diseases as a threat to our soldiers and national security. Our poor and worsening baseline health (and lack of communities that support health) and our increasing vaccine hesitancy put us at even greater risk for the next pandemic than we were for COVID-19. That's why even pre-pandemic, my focus was on mental health, and chronic disease risks like hypertension, and smoking. It's why I was addressing vaccine hesitancy that led to several measles outbreaks in 2019 before my efforts were, ironically, sidetracked by COVID-19. It's why I continue to prioritize these issues in my work, as doing so will help build resilience for whatever crisis hits us next, and it's why I finish this book talking about these issues. Because no matter your political affiliation or who resides at 1600 Pennsylvania Avenue, we seem to continue to ignore and fall victim to the same issues, over and over again. It's like knowing what happened to the *Titanic* and still going out and hitting that same iceberg. Surviving COVID-19 wasn't just about the virus. It was and is about surviving ourselves, our biases, and our failure to address root causes that contributed to our suffering.

We can and must do better.

ENDNOTES

1   "Executive Summary from the Surgeon General's Call to Action to Control
    Hypertension," Office of the Surgeon General, last reviewed October 6, 2020.
    *https://www.hhs.gov/surgeongeneral/reports-and-publications/disease-prevention-
    wellness/hypertension-executive-summary/index.html*

2   Centers for Disease Control and Prevention, "CDC Museum Covid-19
    Timeline," last reviewed March 15, 2023. *https://www.cdc.gov/museum/timeline/
    covid19.html#Early-2020.*

3   Benjamin Mueller, "New Data Links Pandemic's Origins to Raccoon Dogs at
    Wuhan Market," *New York Times,* March 16, 2023. *https://www.nytimes.com/2023/
    03/16/science/covid-wuhan-market-raccoon-dogs-lab-leak.html?searchResultPosition=2*

4   AJMC Staff, "A Timeline of COVID-19 Developments in 2020," AJMC,
    January 1, 2021. *https://www.ajmc.com/view/a-timeline-of-COVID19-
    developments-in-2020*

5   Michael Corkery and Annie Karni, "Trump Administration Restricts
    Entry Into U.S. From China." *New York Times,* January 31, 2020.
    *https://www.nytimes.com/2020/01/31/business/china-travel-coronavirus.
    html?action=click&module=RelatedLinks&pgtype=Article.*

6   Centers for Disease Control and Prevention, "Handwashing in Communities:
    Clean Hands Save Lives—When and How to Wash Your Hands," last
    reviewed November 15, 2022. *https://www.cdc.gov/handwashing/when-how-
    handwashing.html*

7   60 Minutes, "March 2020: Dr. Anthony Fauci Talks with Dr Jon LaPook about
    Covid-19," March 8, 2020, YouTube video, 1:27. *https://www.youtube.com/
    watch?v=PRa6t_e7dgI*

8   Yen Lee Angela Kwok, Jan Gralton, and Mary-Louise McLaws, "Face Touching:
    A Frequent Habit That Has Implications for Hand Hygiene," *American
    Journal of Infection Control* 43, no. 2 (2015): 112–14. *https://doi.org/10.1016/j.
    ajic.2014.10.015*

9   Roni Caryn Rabin and Emily Anthes, "The Virus Is an Airborne Threat, the C.D.C. Acknowledges," *New York Times*, May 7, 2021. *https://www.nytimes. com/2021/05/07/health/coronavirus-airborne-threat.html*

10 Dyani Lewis, "Why the Who Took Two Years to Say Covid Is Airborne," *Nature*, April 6, 2022. *https://www.nature.com/articles/d41586-022-00925-7*

11 Allison McCann, Nadja Popovich, and Jin Wu, "Italy's Virus Shutdown Came Too Late. What Happens Now?" *New York Times*, April 5, 2020. *https://www. nytimes.com/interactive/2020/04/05/world/europe/italy-coronavirus-lockdown-reopen.html*

12 Samantha Kiernan and Madeleine DeVita, "Travel Restrictions on China Due to COVID-19," *Think Global Health*, April 6, 2020. *https://www. thinkglobalhealth.org/article/travel-restrictions-china-due-COVID-19*

13 Lauren J. Tanz, ScD et al., "A Qualitative Assessment of Circumstances Surrounding Drug Overdose Deaths During Early Stages of the COVID-19 Pandemic," Centers for Disease Control and Prevention, SUDORS Data Brief No. 2, August 2022. *https://www.cdc.gov/drugoverdose/databriefs/sudors-2.html*

14 "New Analysis Shows 8% Increase in U.S. Domestic Violence Incidents Following Pandemic Stay-At-Home Orders," Council on Criminal Justice, accessed April 21, 2023. *https://counciloncj.org/new-analysis-shows-8-increase-in-u-s-domestic-violence-incidents-following-pandemic-stay-at-home-orders/*

15 Media Matters for America, from the March 24, 202 edition of Fox News' *Hannity. https://www.mediamatters.org/media/3863991*

16 Jerome Adams, handwritten notes from task force meeting, February 9, 2020.

17 "Seriously people, STOP BUYING MASKS!" tweet by Jerome Adams, March 1, 2020.

18 Emily Tillett and Margaret Brennan, "Former Trump Deputy National Security Adviser Matt Pottinger Details 'Grave Misstep' in Pandemic Response," *CBS News,* February 20, 2021. *https://www.cbsnews.com/news/former-deputy-nsa-matt-pottinger/*

19 Deborah Netburn, "A Timeline of the CDC's Advice on Face Masks," *Los Angeles Times*, July 27, 2021. *https://www.latimes.com/science/story/2021-07-27/timeline-cdc-mask-guidance-during-COVID-19-pandemic*; Deborah L. Birx, *Silent Invasion: The Untold Story of the Trump Administration, Covid-19, and Preventing the Next Pandemic Before It's Too Late* (New York: Harper, 2022).

20 Centers for Disease Control and Prevention, "CDC Museum Covid-19 Timeline." *https://www.cdc.gov/museum/timeline/covid19.html#Early-2020*

21 Elise Reuter, "Watchdog Faults FDA for Rushing COVID-19 Tests to Market by Easing Emergency Use Rules, *MedTechDive*, September 21, 2022. *https://www.medtechdive.com/news/oig-report-fda-eua-COVID-test-problems/632345/*

22 Ibid.

23 CNN, "Tapper Presses Surgeon General: You Can't Even Give Me a Yes or No Answer?," March 8, 2020, YouTube video, 9:42. *https://youtu.be/9nYHBlwgU9A*

24 Lindsey Dawson and Jennifer Kates, "Rapid Home Tests for COVID-19: Issues with Availability and Access in the U.S.," KFF, November 4, 2021. *https://www.kff.org/report-section/rapid-home-tests-for-COVID-19-issues-with-availability-and-access-in-the-u-s-issue-brief/*

25 Jim Frederick, "By the Numbers: How Community Pharmacists Measure Up," *DSN*, March 12, 2015. *https://drugstorenews.com/pharmacy/numbers-how-community-pharmacists-measure#:~:text=Roughly%209-out-of-10%20Americans%20live%20within%20five%20miles%20of,one%20of%20the%20nation's%20biggest%20sources%20of%20employment*

26 Centers for Disease Control and Prevention, "CDC Museum Covid-19 Timeline." *https://www.cdc.gov/museum/timeline/covid19.html#Early-2020*

27 CNN, "'This is rape': Protesters Yell at Parents Walking with Masked Kids at School Event," October 8, 2021, YouTube video, 3:25. *https://youtu.be/JL20TVNGaqc*

28 10 Tampa Bay, "DeSantis Tells Tampa Students to Take Off Face Masks at USF Event," March 2, 2022, YouTube video, 0:25. *https://youtu.be/4CxONX5uNho*

29 MSNBC, "Student Berated by DeSantis Speaks Out | Zerlina," March 4, 2022, YouTube Video, 6:43. *https://youtu.be/YTwa2OlMyvU*

30 CNN, "Tapper presses surgeon general."

31 Ibid.

32 Deidre McPhillips, "People of Color Less Likely to Receive Paxlovid and Other Covid-19 Treatments, According to CDC Study," CNN, October 27, 2022, *https://amp.cnn.com/cnn/2022/10/27/health/paxlovid-prescription-disparities-race-ethnicity/index.html?fbclid=IwAR2chE0gTXorHqRJkfdKAjPnRX_xJYqZUiWM1z0U1gUryLy2RYsJkVruHzQ*

33 Meredith Wadman, "Why COVID-19 Is More Deadly in People with Obesity—Even if They're Young," *Science*, September 8, 2020. *https://www.science.org/content/article/why-COVID-19-more-deadly-people-obesity-even-if-theyre-young*

34 Centers for Disease Control and Prevention, "Obesity and Overweight," last reviewed January 5, 2023. *https://www.cdc.gov/nchs/fastats/obesity-overweight.htm*

35 Joyce Frieden, "Put CDC Back in Charge of Fighting COVID-19, Expert Says," Medpage Today, October 17, 2022. *https://www.medpagetoday.com/infectiousdisease/COVID19vaccine/101263*

36 CNN, "Tapper presses surgeon general."

37 "US Surgeon General Details Spread of Coronavirus and Debate over Masks," interview with Robin Roberts, *Good Morning America*, ABC News, April 1, 2020. *https://abcnews.go.com/GMA/News/video/us-surgeon-general-details-spread-coronavirus-debate-masks-69912642*

38 Robert Kuznia, "The Timetable for a Coronavirus Vaccine Is 18 Months. Experts Say That's Risky," CNN, April 1, 2020. *https://www.cnn.com/2020/03/31/us/coronavirus-vaccine-timetable-concerns-experts-invs/index.html*

39 Reverend Jessie Jackson, personal phone call with author, April 15, 2020.

40 Stephen Feller, "WHO Renames Monkeypox to Avoid Racist, Stigmatizing Connotations," Healio News, November 28, 2022. *https://www.healio.com/news/infectious-disease/20221128/who-renames-monkeypox-to-avoid-racist-stigmatizing-connotations*

41 "WHO Issues Best Practices for Naming New Human Infectious Diseases," World Health Organization, May 8, 2015. *https://www.who.int/news/item/08-05-2015-who-issues-best-practices-for-naming-new-human-infectious-diseases*

42 *Los Angeles Times*, "Trump Calls the Coronavirus the 'Kung Flu,'" June 20, 2020, YouTube video, 2:02. *https://www.youtube.com/watch?v=fN2tgtcKGck*

43 "US Surgeon General Jerome Adams on Coronavirus: 'This Week It's Going to Get Bad'| TODAY," March 23, 2020, YouTube video, 8:18. *https://youtu.be/F_JfmcHlziA*

44 Ibid.

45 Zacks Equity Research, "Stock Market News for Mar 23, 2020," Yahoo! Finance, March 23, 2020. *https://finance.yahoo.com/news/stock-market-news-mar-23-133301437.html*

46   Frank Vogl, "March 23, 2020: The Day the US Economy Did Not Crash," *The Globalist*, May 14, 2020. *https://www.theglobalist.com/united-states-stock-market-wall-street-federal-reserve-unemployment-inequality-financial-crisis/*

47   Emily Cochrane and Nicholas Fandos, "Top Senate Democrat and Treasury Secretary Say They Are Near a Stimulus Deal," *New York Times*, March 23, 2020. *https://www.nytimes.com/2020/03/23/us/politics/stimulus-package-for-coronavirus.html?searchResultPosition=11*

48   NAACP president Derrick Johnson, personal phone call with author, April 2020.

49   Nia Malika-Henderson, "Cousin Pookie Is Back! And Yes, He Is Still Sitting on the Couch," *Washington Post*, October 20, 2014. *https://www.washingtonpost.com/news/the-fix/wp/2014/10/20/cousin-pookie-is-back-and-yes-he-is-still-sitting-on-the-couch/*

50   Fox Business, "Trump, Coronavirus Task Force Hold Press Briefing at White House | 4/10/2020," livestream on April 10, 2020, YouTube video, 2:14:28. *https://www.youtube.com/watch?v=c5F9vPFphmQ*

51   Charlie Nash, "AOC: Surgeon General Only Brought Up Personal Responsibility on Coronavirus 'When We Started Talking About Black Americans,'" *Mediaite,* April 15, 2020.

52   Maxine Waters, "Donald Trump has found a new vessel by which to spew his racist dog whistles: his Surgeon General Jerome Adams…," Facebook, April 13, 2020. *https://www.facebook.com/MaxineWaters/*

53   US Department of Health and Human Services, "Smoking Cessation: A Report of the Surgeon General," US Department of Health and Human Services, Centers for Disease Control and Prevention, National Center for Chronic Disease Prevention and Health Promotion, Office on Smoking and Health, (Atlanta, GA: 2020), accessed April 21, 2023. *https://www.hhs.gov/sites/default/files/2020-cessation-sgr-full-report.pdf*

54   "Tobacco Use in Racial and Ethnic Populations," American Lung Association, last updated November 17, 2022. *https://www.lung.org/quit-smoking/smoking-facts/impact-of-tobacco-use/tobacco-use-racial-and-ethnic*; US Department of Health and. Human Services, "Smoking Cessation – 2020."

55 Dan Diamond, "Surgeon General Gets Pushed to Sidelines, Sparking Questions," *Politico,* April 20, 2020. *https://www.politico.com/news/2020/04/20/surgeon-general-coronavirus-197508*

56 Curtis Bunn, "Black Health Experts Say Surgeon General's Comments Reflect Lack of Awareness of Black Community," NBC News, April 15, 2020. *https://www.nbcnews.com/news/nbcblk/Black-health-experts-say-surgeon-general-s-comments-reflect-lack-n1183711*

57 NAACP president Derrick Johnson, personal phone call with author on April 10th, 2020.

58 Oprah, personal phone call with author.

59 Nick Gass, "Trump on Small Hands: 'I Guarantee You There's No Problem,'" *Politico,* March 3, 2016. *https://www.politico.com/blogs/2016-gop-primary-live-updates-and-results/2016/03/donald-trump-small-hands-220223*

60 The Associated Press, "Donald Trump Criticizes Hillary Clinton," *New York Times,* October 2, 2016, video, 1:02. *https://www.nytimes.com/video/us/elections/100000004685807/donald-trump-criticizes-hillary-clinton.html?searchResultPosition=1*

61 Marc Caputo and Christopher Cadelago, "Dems Warm to Biden's Bunker Strategy," *Politico,* June 24, 2020. *https://www.politico.com/news/2020/06/24/dems-warm-to-bidens-bunker-strategy-338853*

62 Tim Malloy and Doug Schwartz, "Biden Holds 11 Point Lead as Trump Approval on Coronavirus Dips, Quinnipiac University National Poll Finds; Almost Half Say Second Wave of Coronavirus 'Very Likely' in Fall," Quinnipiac University / Poll, released May 20, 2020. *https://poll.qu.edu/images/polling/us/us05202020_ugjm33.pdf*

63 Howard, Matt C., "Personality and Individual Differences," U.S. National Library of Medicine, February 15, 2021. *https://www.ncbi.nlm.nih.gov/pmc/articles/PMC7543707/#:~:text=Men%20were%20more%20likely%20to%20perceive%20face%20masks,mask%2C%20it%20does%20relate%20to%20face%20mask%20perceptions.*

64 Richard V. Reeves and Beyond Deng, "At least 65,000 More Men than Woman Have Died from COVID-19 in the US," Brookings, October 19, 2021. *https://www.brookings.edu/blog/up-front/2021/10/19/at-least-65000-more-men-than-women-have-died-from-COVID-19-in-the-us/*; Juan Siliezar, "Why Do

More Men Die of COVID? It's Likely Not What You Think," *The Harvard Gazette*, January 20, 2022. *https://news.harvard.edu/gazette/story/2022/01/harvard-study-looks-at-COVID-19-sex-disparities/*

65   Sean Neumann, "Rep. Maxine Waters Draws Republican Backlash for 'Confrontational' Comment but Says She Was 'Distorted,'" Yahoo News, April 19, 2021. *https://news.yahoo.com/rep-maxine-waters-draws-republican-204105511.html*

66   "Joe Biden Would Use Federal Power to Require Face Masks in Public If Elected: 'These Masks Make a Gigantic Difference,'" CBS News Pittsburgh, June 25, 2020. *https://www.cbsnews.com/pittsburgh/news/joe-biden-talks-face-masks-coronavirus-and-rallies/*

67   Today, "Surgeon General Jerome Adams: If You Go Out For July 4, Wear A Mask | TODAY," July 3, 2020, YouTube video, 5:10. *https://youtu.be/JCncn41-xlk*

68   Ibid.

69   D. L. Hughley, and Doug Moe, *How to Survive America* (NY: HarperCollins, 2021), pp 11–14.

70   Larry Buchanan, Quoctrung Bui, and Jugal K. Patel, "Black Lives Matter May Be the Largest Movement in U.S. History," *New York Times*, July 3, 2020. *https://www.nytimes.com/interactive/2020/07/03/us/george-floyd-protests-crowd-size.html*

71   Julia Ries, "Experts Say COVID-19 Is Airborne: Here's How You Can Stay Safe," Healthline, October 7, 2020. *https://www.healthline.com/health-news/experts-say-COVID-19-is-airborne-heres-how-you-can-stay-safe*

72   "Asthma and African Americans," US Department of Health and Human Services Office of Minority Health, last updated February 17, 2023. *https://minorityhealth.hhs.gov/omh/browse.aspx?lvl=4&lvlid=15*

73   Goyal, Monika K et al., "Racial Disparities in Pain Management of Children with Appendicitis in Emergency Departments," *JAMA Pediatrics* vol. 169,11 (2015): 996-1002. doi:10.1001/jamapediatrics.2015.1915, *https://pubmed.ncbi.nlm.nih.gov/26366984/*

74   "Working Together to Reduce Black Maternal Mortality," Centers for Disease Control and Prevention, last reviewed April 3, 2023. *https://www.cdc.gov/healthequity/features/maternal-mortality/index.html*

75 "Facts about Hypertension," Centers for Disease Control and Prevention, last reviewed January 5, 2023. *https://www.cdc.gov/bloodpressure/facts.htm*

76 Khiara M. Bridges, "Implicit Bias and Racial Disparities in Health Care," American Bar Association. *https://www.americanbar.org/groups/crsj/publications/ human_rights_magazine_home/the-state-of-healthcare-in-the-united-states/ racial-disparities-in-health-care/*

77 Dan Diamond, "U.S. Surgeon General: George Floyd 'Could Have Been Me,'" June 11, 2020, *Politico*'s Pulse Check, produced by Jenny Ament, Irene Nogushi, and Annie Rees, podcast, 29:51, https://politicos-pulse-check. simplecast.com/episodes/that-could-have-been-me-08spWlKd

78 "Fatal Police Shootings of Unarmed Black People in US More than 3 Times as High as in Whites," BMJ, accessed April 21, 2023. *https://www.bmj.com/ company/newsroom/fatal-police-shootings-of-unarmed-black-people-in-us-more- than-3-times-as-high-as-in-whites/*; "Mapping Police Violence," Mapping Police Violence, last updated February 28, 2023. *https://mappingpoliceviolence.org*

79 "Health Equity and Flu," Centers for Disease Control and Prevention, last reviewed October 18, 2022 . *https://www.cdc.gov/flu/highrisk/disparities-racial- ethnic-minority-groups.html*

80 Crystal Grant, "Algorithms Are Making Decisions about Health Care, Which May Only Worsen Medical Racism," ACLU, October 3, 2022. *https://www.aclu. org/news/privacy-technology/algorithms-in-health-care-may-worsen-medical-racism*

81 Usha Lee McFarling, "Inaccurate Pulse Oximeter Readings Tied to Less Supplemental Oxygen for Darker-Skinned ICU Patients," *STAT,* July 11, 2022. *https://www.statnews.com/2022/07/11/inaccurate-pulse-oximeter-readings-tied-to- less-supplemental-oxygen-for-darker-skinned-icu-patients/*

82 Hannah Gaskill, "Judge Weighing Motion to Dismiss Henrietta Lacks' Family Lawsuit Against Biotech Firm," Maryland Matters, May 17, 2022. *https://www. marylandmatters.org/2022/05/17/judge-weighing-motion-to-dismiss-henrietta-lacks- family-lawsuit-against-biotech-firm/#:~:text=According%20to%20Benjamin%20 L.,companies%20since%20they%20were%20harvested*

83 Kenny Cooper, "Old Wounds Reopen After Report Details Mishandling of Remains of MOVE Bombing Victims," October 5, 2022, in *Morning Edition*, podcast. *https://www.npr.org/2022/10/05/1126885171/old-wounds-reopen-after- report-details-mishandling-of-remains-of-move-bombing-vi*; Michael Levenson,

"Decades After Police Bombing, Philadelphians 'Sickened' by Handling of Victim's Bones," *New York Times*, last updated May 15, 2021. *https://www.nytimes.com/2021/04/24/us/move-rowhouse-bombing-victim-remains.html*

84   Kristina Fiore, "Black Doctor Who Died of COVID Said Racism Impacted Care," Medpage Today, December 23, 2020. *https://www.medpagetoday.com/infectiousdisease/COVID19/90412*

85   Marina Del Rios et al., "Covid-19 Is an Inverse Equity Story, Not a Racial Equity Success Story," *STAT*, October 25, 2022. *https://www.statnews.com/2022/10/25/COVID-19-inverse-equity-story-not-racial-equity-success-story/*

86   Ibid.

87   Ibid.

88   Usha Lee McFarling, "After 40 Years, Medical Schools Are Admitting Fewer Black Male or Native American Students," *STAT*, April 28, 2021. *https://www.statnews.com/2021/04/28/medical-schools-admitting-fewer-black-male-or-native-american-students/*

89   Ibid.

90   Black Men in White Coats. accessed April 23, 2023. *https://www.blackmeninwhitecoats.org/*

91   Usha Lee McFarling, "'It Was Stolen from Me': Black Doctors Are Forced Out of Training Programs at Far Higher Rates than White Residents," *STAT*, June 20, 2022. *https://www.statnews.com/2022/06/20/black-doctors-forced-out-of-training-programs-at-far-higher-rates-than-white-residents/*

92   Jared Leone, "Coronavirus: City Fills Skatepark with 37 Tons of Sand to Deter Skaters," KIRO7, April 18, 2020. *https://www.kiro7.com/news/trending/coronavirus-city-fills-skatepark-with-37-tons-sand-deter-skaters/P36K2J3RLBBCZB3RVJC3G2X5HY/*

93   Allyson Blair, "HPD Suspends COVID-19 Enforcement Patrols after Audit Finds Major Overtime Violations," *Hawaii News Now*, November 20, 2020. *https://www.hawaiinewsnow.com/2020/11/20/hpd-suspends-COVID-enforcement-patrols-after-audit-finds-major-overtime-violations/*

94   Rosemarie Bernardo, "New Prosecutor Wants Surgeon General's Case Dismissed," *Star Advertiser*, January 20, 2021. *https://www.staradvertiser.com/2021/01/20/hawaii-news/new-prosecutor-wants-surgeon-generals-case-dismissed/*

95 Rick Daysog, "Nearly 60,000 Citations Issued for Violating Emergency Orders Thrown Out," Hawaii News Now, November 24, 2020. *https://www.hawaiinewsnow.com/2020/11/23/more-than-citations-issued-violating-emergency-orders-have-been-thrown-out/*

96 Ibid.

97 "Educational Instituations," National Center for Education Statistics, accessed April 23, 2023. *https://nces.ed.gov/fastfacts/display.asp?id=84;* Imed Bouchrika, PhD, "75 U.S. College Statistics: 2023 Facts, Data & Trends," *Research.com,* April 20, 2023. *https://research.com/universities-colleges/college-statistics*

98 "Schools and Staffing Survey (SASS)," National Center for Education Statistics, accessed April 21, 2023. *https://nces.ed.gov/surveys/sass/tables/sass1112_2013314_t1s_002.asp*

99 Rhitu Chatterjee, "Nearly 8 Million Kids Lost a Parent or Primary Caregiver to the Pandemic," September 6, 2022, in *Goats and Soda, Stories of Life in a Changing World,* podcast. *https://www.npr.org/sections/goatsandsoda/2022/09/06/1121254016/nearly-8-million-kids-lost-a-parent-or-primary-caregiver-to-the-pandemic*

100 "Schools," ASCE's 2021 Infrastructure Report Card, July 12, 2022. *https://infrastructurereportcard.org/cat-item/schools-infrastructure/*

101 Michael Hiltzik, "Column: Did Sweden Beat the Pandemic Refusing to Lock Down? No, Its Record Is Disastrous," *Los Angeles Times,* March 31, 2022. *https://www.latimes.com/business/story/2022-03-31/sweden-COVID-policy-was-a-disaster*

102 "Dr. Birx: Trump Presented Graphs that I Never Made," CNN Business, video, 1:46. *https://www.cnn.com/videos/media/2021/01/24/deborah-birx-trump-coronavirus-briefings-rs-vpx.cnn*

103 Simone Pathe, "Marcy Kaptur Breaks New Record in Congress with a Familiar Warning to the Democratic Party," CNN Politics, January 7, 2023. *https://www.cnn.com/2023/01/07/politics/marcy-kaptur-longest-serving-woman-congress/index.html*

104 "Los Angeles County Population vs. State Populations," *Los Angeles Almanac,* accessed April 21, 2023. *https://www.laalmanac.com/population/po04a.php*

105 Carl Smith, "Assessing the Global COVID Response: Hard Lessons for the U.S.," *Governing,* September 21, 2022. *https://www.governing.com/now/assessing-the-global-COVID-response-hard-lessons-for-the-u-s*

106 "Is it true? Can COVID-19 vaccines alter my DNA?," Australian Government – Department of Health and Aged Care, last updated May 10, 2022. *https://www.health.gov.au/our-work/COVID-19-vaccines/is-it-true/is-it-true-can-COVID-19-vaccines-alter-my-dna*

107 Steven Salzberg, "De-platform The Disinformation Dozen," *Forbes,* July 19, 2021. *https://www.forbes.com/sites/stevensalzberg/2021/07/19/de-platform-the-disinformation-dozen/?sh=2576a2847378*

108 "Confronting Health Misinformation: The U.S. Surgeon General's Advisory on Building a Healthy Information Environment," Surgeon General's Advisory, 2021. Accessed April 21, 2023. *https://www.hhs.gov/sites/default/files/surgeon-general-misinformation-advisory.pdf*

109 C-SPAN, "Vice Presidential Debate between Mike Pence and Kamala Harris," livestream on October 7, 2020, YouTube video, 1:46:08. *https://youtu.be/t_G0ia3JOVs*

110 Bob Woodward, *Rage,* (New York: Simon & Schuster, 2020), pp. 233–238.

111 "Gov. Cuomo: 'I'm Not Going to Trust the Federal Government's Opinion' on Potential Approved COVID-19 Vaccine," CBS News, September 25, 2020. *https://www.cbsnews.com/newyork/news/cuomo-vaccine-covid/*

112 "Whoopi Goldberg Receives COVID-19 Vaccine," ABC News, March 11, 2021, video, 2:44. *https://abcnews.go.com/theview/video/whoopi-goldberg-receives-COVID-19-vaccine-76393629*

113 Cara Buckley, "Tyler Perry Gets COVID Vaccine on TV to Reassure Black Skeptics," *New York Times,* updated January 30, 2021. *https://www.nytimes.com/2021/01/28/arts/tyler-perry-COVID-vaccine-skeptics.html*

114 Arek Sarkissian, "Desantis Says Florida Is 'Affirmatively Against' Covid-19 Vaccines for Young Kids," *Yahoo! News,* June 16, 2022. *https://news.yahoo.com/desantis-says-florida-affirmatively-against-165949732.html?guccounter=1*; Nicholas Reimann, "DeSantis Changes Mind—Allows Florida To Buy Covid Vaccines For Kids 5 And Younger," *Forbes,* June 17, 2022. *https://www.forbes.com/sites/nicholasreimann/2022/06/17/desantis-changes-mind-allows-florida-to-buy-COVID-vaccines-for-kids-5-and-younger-report-says/?sh=1d8a015b3b83*; Arek Sarkissian, "Desantis Says Florida Is 'Affirmatively Against' Covid-19 Vaccines for Young Kids," *Politico,* June 16, 2022. *https://www.politico.com/news/2022/06/16/desantis-COVID-vaccine-florida-kids-fda-00040191*

115 "Child and Adolescent Mortality," ChildStats Forum on Child and Family Statistics, *America's Children in Brief: Key National Indicators of Well-Being, 2022*, accessed April 21, 2023. *https://www.childstats.gov/americaschildren/mortality.asp*

116 James Lawler, MD, quote. Author's personal conversation with James Lawler, December 1, 2022.

117 Peng Gao, Jue Liu, and Min Liu, "Effect of Covid-19 Vaccines on Reducing the Risk of Long COVID in the Real World: A Systematic Review and Meta-Analysis," *International Journal of Environmental Research and Public Health* 19, no. 19 (2022): 12422. *https://doi.org/10.3390/ijerph191912422*

118 "Long COVID or Post-COVID Conditions," Centers for Disease Control and Prevention, updated December 16, 2022. *https://www.cdc.gov/coronavirus/2019-ncov/long-term-effects/index.html*

119 Jen Christensen, "Long Covid Responsible for Thousands of US Deaths, Report Says, but True Numbers Are Likely Much Higher," CNN, December 14, 2022. *https://www.cnn.com/2022/12/14/health/long-COVID-deaths/index.html*

120 Pien Huang, "How Monoclonal Antibodies Lost the Fight with New COVID Variants," November 20, 2022, in *Morning Edition*, podcast. *https://www.npr.org/sections/health-shots/2022/11/20/1137892932/monoclonal-antibodies-COVID-treatment*

121 Peter Loftus and Melanie Grayce West, "First Covid-19 Vaccine Given to U.S. Public," *Wall Street Journal*, December 14, 2020. *https://www.supremecourt.gov/opinions/urls_cited/ot2021/21a90/21a90-1.pdf*

122 Ibid.

123 Ken Alltucker, "'Medication I Can't Live Without': Lupus Patients Struggle to Get Hydroxychloroquine, in Demand for COVID-19," *USA Today*, updated April 19, 2020, *https://www.usatoday.com/story/news/health/2020/04/18/hydroxychloroquine-coronavirus-creates-shortage-lupus-drug/5129896002/*

124 Dave Roos, "How Crude Smallpox Inoculations Helped George Washington Win the War," *History*, updated May 18, 2020. *https://www.history.com/news/smallpox-george-washington-revolutionary-war*

125 "Influenza Vaccine Mandates for Child Care and Pre-K August 2020," *Immunize.org*, updated on February 28, 2022. *https://www.immunize.org/laws/flu_childmap.pdf*

126 Lissandra Villa, "The Pandemic Is Causing a Shortage of Poll Workers. Can States Recruit Enough by Election Day?," *TIME*, August 5, 2020. *https://time.com/5876195/coronavirus-poll-workers-election/*

127 Martin Pengelly, "Trump Administration Removes Obama Surgeon General Pick Vivek Murthy," *The Guardian*, April 22, 2017. *https://www.theguardian.com/us-news/2017/apr/22/trump-administration-removes-surgeon-general-vivek-murthy*

128 Dr. Vivek Murthy, private phone call with author.

129 Carl Zimmer, "U.S. Is Blind to Contagious New Virus Variant, Scientists Warn," *New York Times*, January 6, 2021. *https://www.nytimes.com/2021/01/06/health/coronavirus-variant-tracking.html?searchResultPosition=24*

130 Pam Belluck, "He Was Hospitalized for Covid-19. Then Hospitalized Again. And Again.," *New York Times*, December 30, 2020. *https://www.nytimes.com/2020/12/30/health/COVID-hospital-readmissions.html?searchResultPosition=1*

131 John Bowden, "Biden says as president he would keep Fauci," *The Hill*, June 30, 2020. *https://thehill.com/homenews/campaign/505319-biden-says-as-president-he-would-keep-fauci/*

132 Sharon Weinberge and Jana Winter, "Biden says the Trump White House won't give him COVID stockpile information. Here it is." *Yahoo News*, November 18, 2020. *https://uk.movies.yahoo.com/biden-says-trump-white-house-wont-give-him-covid-stockpile-information-002027031.html*

133 "Transcript of Alyssa Farah Griffin's Interview with House January 6 Committee," contributed by CNN Digital, released December 29, 2022. *https://www.documentcloud.org/documents/23558377-transcript-of-alyssa-farah-griffins-interview-with-house-january-6-committee*

134 Charlie McCarthy, "Jerome Adams Claims HHS Won't Verify His Employment as Surgeon General," *Newsmax*, September 22, 2021. *https://www.newsmax.com/politics/surgeon-general-jerome-adams-hhs-employment/2021/09/22/id/1037460/*

135 "Hillary Clinton: 'Trump Knows He's an Illegitimate President,'" interview by Jane Pauley, *Sunday Morning*, CBS News, September 29, 2019, video. *https://www.cbsnews.com/video/hillary-clinton-trump-knows-hes-an-illegitimate-president/*

136 "National Academy of Medicine Elects 100 New Members," National Academy of Medicine, October 18, 2021. *https://nam.edu/national-academy-of-medicine-elects-100-new-members-2021/*

137 Arthur Lupia, "Political Endorsements Can Affect Scientific Credibility," *Nature,* March 20, 2023. *https://www.nature.com/articles/d41586-023-00799-3*

138 Megha Kaveri, "Hybrid Immunity Protects Better Against Hospitalisation and Severe Covid Infection," *Health Policy Watch,* January 19, 2023. *https:// healthpolicy-watch.news/covid-hybrid-immunity-better/*

139 Shishira Sreenivas, "What to Know About Vitamin D and COVID-19," *WebMD,* January 2, 2023. *https://www.webmd.com/lung/vitamin-d-COVID-19-what-to-know*

140 "Executive Summary from the Surgeon General's Call to Action to Control Hypertension," Office of the Surgeon General, last reviewed October 6, 2020. *https://www.hhs.gov/surgeongeneral/reports-and-publications/disease-prevention-wellness/hypertension-executive-summary/index.html*

141 Manuel Roig-Franzia, "Surgeon General Jerome Adams May Be the Nicest Guy in the Trump Administration. But Is That What America Needs Right Now?" *Washington Post,* July 12, 2020. *https://www.washingtonpost.com/lifestyle/style/ surgeon-general-jerome-adams-may-be-the-nicest-guy-in-the-trump-administration-but-is-that-what-america-needs-right-now/2020/07/11/39529cec-a1c1-11ea-9590-1858a893bd59_story.html*

142 Mike Snider, "First At-Home Combination Test for Covid and Flu Authorized by FDA," *USA Today,* February 25, 2023. *https://www.usatoday.com/story/news/ health/2023/02/25/first-covid-flu-home-test-authorized-fda/11347202002/*

143 Permanente, Kaiser. "Saving Lives: Study Finds That Paxlovid Reduces Risk of COVID-19 Hospitalization and Death by 90%." *SciTechDaily,* 3 May 2023, *scitechdaily.com/saving-lives-study-finds-that-paxlovid-reduces-risk-of-covid-19-hospitalization-and-death-by-90/*

144 Adam Rogers, "Could a Janky, Jury-Rigged Air Purifier Help Fight Covid-19?," *Wired,* August 6, 2020. *https://www.wired.com/story/ could-a-janky-jury-rigged-air-purifier-help-fight-COVID-19/*

145 Associated Press, "Utah Jazz Star Center Rudy Gobert Tests Positive for COVID-19," ESPN, January 6, 2022. *https://www.espn.com/nba/story/_/ id/33008714/utah-jazz-star-center-ruday-gobert-tests-positive-COVID-19*

146 Sam Quinn, "Rudy Gobert Says He Still Isn't Fully Recovered from Covid-19," CBS Sports, June 28, 2020. *https://www.cbssports.com/nba/news/ rudy-gobert-says-he-still-isnt-fully-recovered-from-covid-19/*

147 Janie Haseman and Aleszu Bajak, "COVID And Kids: How the
Omicron Surge Is Impacting Child Hospitalizations, School Safety," *USA
Today*, updated January 13, 2022. *https://www.usatoday.com/in-depth/
graphics/2022/01/13/COVID-19-kids-cases-deaths-and-hospitalization-
omcrion-data-charts/9118848002/*; Associated Press, "COVID
Hospitalizations Soar for Kids Under Five," *USA Today*, January 7, 2022,
video, 1:19. *https://www.usatoday.com/videos/news/nation/2022/01/07/
COVID-hospitalizations-soar-kids-under-five/9135052002/*

148 Martha Bellisle and Terry Tang, "US children hospitalized with COVID in record
numbers," *Associated Press*, December 30, 2021. *https://apnews.com/article/coronavirus-
pandemic-health-pandemics-seattle-centers-for-disease-control-and-prevention-75a48
388d6ca85ad88de300f32bfdec6*

149 Andrea Hsu, "Millions of Americans Have Long Covid. Many of Them Are No
Longer Working," July 31, 2022, in *Weekend Edition Sunday*, NPR, podcast.
*https://www.npr.org/2022/07/31/1114375163/long-covid-longhaulers-disability-
labor-ada*

150 Sarah Owermohle, "On the Campaign Trail, Republicans Ramp Up Anti-Science,
Anti-Covid, Often Anti-Fauci Messaging," *STAT*, October 25, 2022. *https://
www.statnews.com/2022/10/25/republicans-campaign-anti-science-anti-fauci/*

151 Farida B. Ahmad MPH, Jodi A. Cisewski MPH, and Robert Anderson PhD,
"Provisional Mortality Data—United States 2021," *Morbidity and Mortality
Weekly Report 2022*; 71:597-600 Centers for Disease Control, updated April 29,
2022. *https://www.cdc.gov/mmwr/volumes/71/wr/mm7117e1.htm*

152 David Wallace-Wells, "How the West Lost COVID," *New York Magazine*,
March 15, 2021. *https://nymag.com/intelligencer/2021/03/how-the-west-lost-
covid-19.html*

153 Benjamin Mueller and Eleanor Lutz, "U.S. Has Far Higher Covid Death Rate
Than Other Wealthy Countries," *New York Times*, February 1, 2022. *https://
www.nytimes.com/interactive/2022/02/01/science/covid-deaths-united-states.html*

154 David Wallace-Wells, "9 Pandemic Narratives We're Getting Wrong," *New York
Times*, January 4, 2023. *https://www.nytimes.com/2023/01/04/opinion/covid-
pandemic-history.html*

155 Adelle M. Banks, "CeCe Winans: 'Absolutely not' paid for COVID-
19 PSA requested by Trump administration," *Religion News*

Service, September 29, 2020. *https://religionnews.com/2020/09/29/cece-winans-absolutely-not-paid-for-psa-requested-by-trump-administration/*

156 Janet W. Lee, "Dennis Quaid, CeCe Winans Claim Coronavirus Interviews Are 'Not Political at All,'" *Variety,* September 26, 2020. *https://variety.com/2020/politics/news/donald-trump-coronavirus-ad-dennis-quaid-cece-winans-1234784767/*; Dennis Quaid (@dennisquaid), "No good deed goes unpoliticized," Instagram video, September 26, 2020. *https://www.instagram.com/p/CFnPi4gB_Gq/?utm_source=ig_embed&utm_campaign=embed_video_watch_again*

157 Andrew Desilver, "U.S. Students' Academic Achievement Still Lags That of Their Peers in Many Other Countries," Pew Research Center, February 15, 2017. *https://www.pewresearch.org/fact-tank/2017/02/15/u-s-students-internationally-math-science/*

158 "Literacy Statistics," *ThinkImpact,* accessed April 21, 2023. *https://www.thinkimpact.com/literacy-statistics/#3-adult-literacy-statistics*

159 Brian Deer, "Andrew Wakefield: the fraud investigation," Brian Deer, accessed April 21, 2023. *https://briandeer.com/mmr/lancet-summary.htm*

160 "My WordPress Blog," *Association of Diversity,* accessed May 16, 2023 *associationofdiversity.org/*

161 Jane Greenhalgh and Selena Simmons-Duffin, "Life expectancy in the U.S. continues to drop, driven by COVID-19," NPR, August 31, 2022. *https://www.npr.org/sections/health-shots/2022/08/31/1120192583/life-expectancy-in-the-u-s-continues-to-drop-driven-by-COVID 19*

162 "Nearly One in Five American Adults Who Have Had COVID-19 Still Have 'Long COVID,'" Centers for Disease Control and Prevention, last reviewed June 22, 2022. *https://www.cdc.gov/nchs/pressroom/nchs_press_releases/2022/20220622.htm*

163 Greg Iacurci, "Millions suffer from long Covid — And It Costs Them $9,000 a Year in Health-Care Expenses, on Average," CNBC, Updated December 9, 2022. *https://www.cnbc.com/2022/12/01/long-COVID-costs-patients-an-average-9000-a-year-in-medical-expenses.html*

164 Jerome Adams, "As Trump's surgeon general, I saw national problems that helped the COVID pandemic spread," *USA Today,* March 30,

2022. *https://www.usatoday.com/story/opinion/contributors/2022/03/30/COVID-pandemic-trump-cdc-surgeon-general/7167537001/?gnt-cfr=1*

165 "Where Does Our Data Come From?," Centers for Disease Control and Prevention, last reviewed January 5, 2023. *https://www.cdc.gov/surveillance/projects/dmi-initiative/where_does_our_data_come_from.html*

166 Alice Park, "Dr. Rochelle Walensky Knows the CDC Made 'Dramatic Mistakes.' Now She's Trying to Fix Them," *TIME*, August 23, 2022. *https://time.com/6207887/cdc-COVID-19-revamp-rochelle-walensky-interview/*

167 Li-Kai Chen, Emma Dorn, Jimmy Sarakatsannis, and Anna Wiesinger, "Teacher Survey: Learning Loss Is Global—and Significant," McKinsey & Company, March 1, 2021. *https://www.mckinsey.com/industries/education/our-insights/teacher-survey-learning-loss-is-global-and-significant*

168 A Joint UNESCO, UNICEF, and World Bank Report, "The State of the Global Education Crisis: A Path to Recovery," The World Bank, UNESCO, and UNICEF, December 3, 2021, p. 6. *https://www.unicef.org/media/111621/file/%20The%20State%20of%20the%20Global%20Education%20Crisis.pdf%20.pdf*

169 *Community Health and Economic Prosperity: Engaging Businesses as Stewards and Stakeholders—A Report of the Surgeon General*, US Department of Health & Human Services, released January 19, 2021. *https://www.hhs.gov/surgeongeneral/reports-and-publications/community-health-economic-prosperity/index.html*

170 "WHO Coronavirus (COVID-19) Dashboard," World Health Organization, accessed April 21, 2023. https://COVID19.who.int/?mapFilter=cases

171 Ibid.

ACKNOWLEDGMENTS

MY ENTIRE FAMILY, INCLUDING MY mother, Edrena, and father, Richard, brothers, Tee and Phillip, and sister, Latoya, and my in laws, Ked and Shelley.

Nancy Peske, who assisted greatly with the writing and editing of this book.

The staff in the office of the surgeon general, including RADM Erica Schwartz, LCDR Dennis Anderson-Villaluz, Lieutenant, CDR Kate Migliaccio-Grabill, CDR Courtney Gustin, LCDR Fengyee Zhou, Capt Joel Dulaigh, Dolly Moorhead, Dr. Janet Wright, Rafael Campos, Amber Channer, Kana Enomoto, and Rochelle Rollins.

All at HHS who supported me, including secretary, Alex Azar, CMS Director Seema Verma, FDA Commissioner, Scott Gottlieb, and RADM Sylvia Trent-Adams.

Mike and Karen Pence.

The staff at CDC, including RADM Anne Schuchat, RADM Wanda Barfield, and Dr. Deb Houry.

The members of the public health service commissioned corps.

The members of the COVID-19 task force, including Dr. Deb Birx, Dr. Tony Fauci, Dr. Bob Redfield, Dr. Steve Hahn, and Admiral Brett Giroir.

The national institutes of health, including Director Francis Collins and NIDA Director Dr. Nora Volkow.

ACL Commissioner, Lance Robertson.

ONDCP Director Jim Carroll.

HUD Secretary Ben Carson.

The people at Indian health services, including Director RADM Michael Weahkee.

General Colin Powell, General Gustav Perna, Oprah Winfrey and Gayle King, Dr. Virginia Caine, Dr: Patrice Harris, Dr. David Satcher, Dr. Eric Barker, Jan Miller, Mike and Karen Pence, Mitch Daniels, Eric Holcomb, Dr. Freeman Hrabowski, Stephanie Bates, Dr. Andrew Trobridge, Chef Jose Andres, the American Society of Anesthesiologists, The Indiana Society of Anesthesiologists, the National Medical Association, the American Medical Association, and the Indiana State Medical Association.

My former team at the Indiana state department of health, including Eric Miller, Tami Barrett, Dr. Jennifer Sullivan, Dr. Joan Duwve, Jennifer O'Malley, and Pam Pontones.

The Association of State and Territorial Health Officers, including Dr. Nicole Alexander-Scott, Dr. Nirav Shah, Dr. Monica Bharel, and Michael Fraser.